28 DAY   ANTI

INFLAMMATORY

DIET BOOK

Simple recipes to stop inflammation, optimize gut health and reduce chronic pain

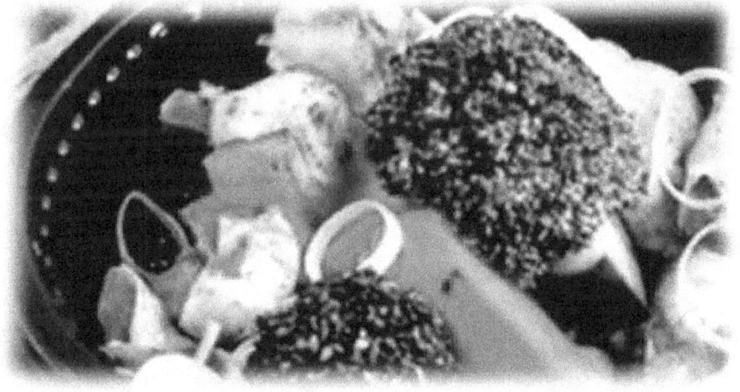

Dr. Grace Hester

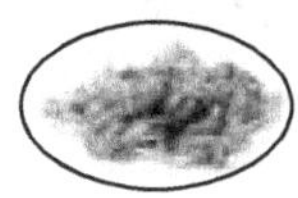 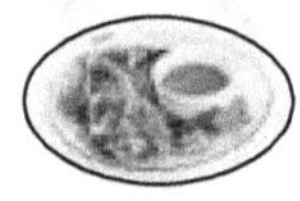 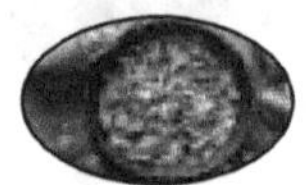

Copyright Page

Disclaimer: The recipes contained in this cookbook are intended for personal use and enjoyment. The author and publisher are not responsible for any health issues or allergic reactions that may arise from the use of the ingredients or recipes provided. It is recommended that individuals with specific dietary concerns or restrictions consult a qualified healthcare professional.

DR. GRACE HESTER

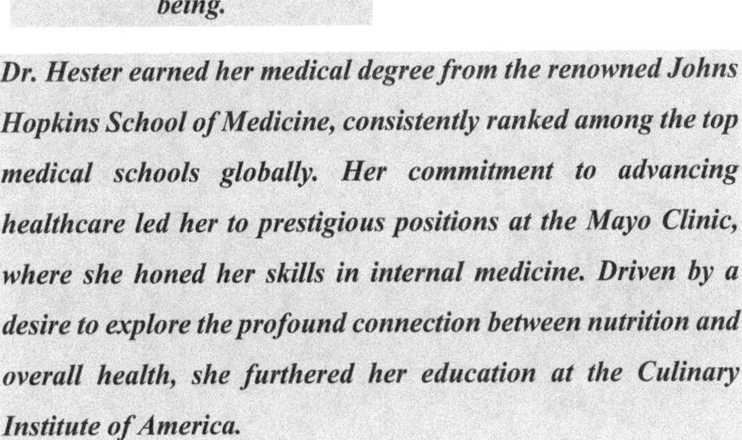

Dr. Grace Hester stands at the intersection of health, passion, and culinary excellence. A distinguished medical professional and accomplished nutritionist, she seamlessly weaves together her expertise to create a holistic approach to well-being.

Dr. Hester earned her medical degree from the renowned Johns Hopkins School of Medicine, consistently ranked among the top medical schools globally. Her commitment to advancing healthcare led her to prestigious positions at the Mayo Clinic, where she honed her skills in internal medicine. Driven by a desire to explore the profound connection between nutrition and overall health, she furthered her education at the Culinary Institute of America.

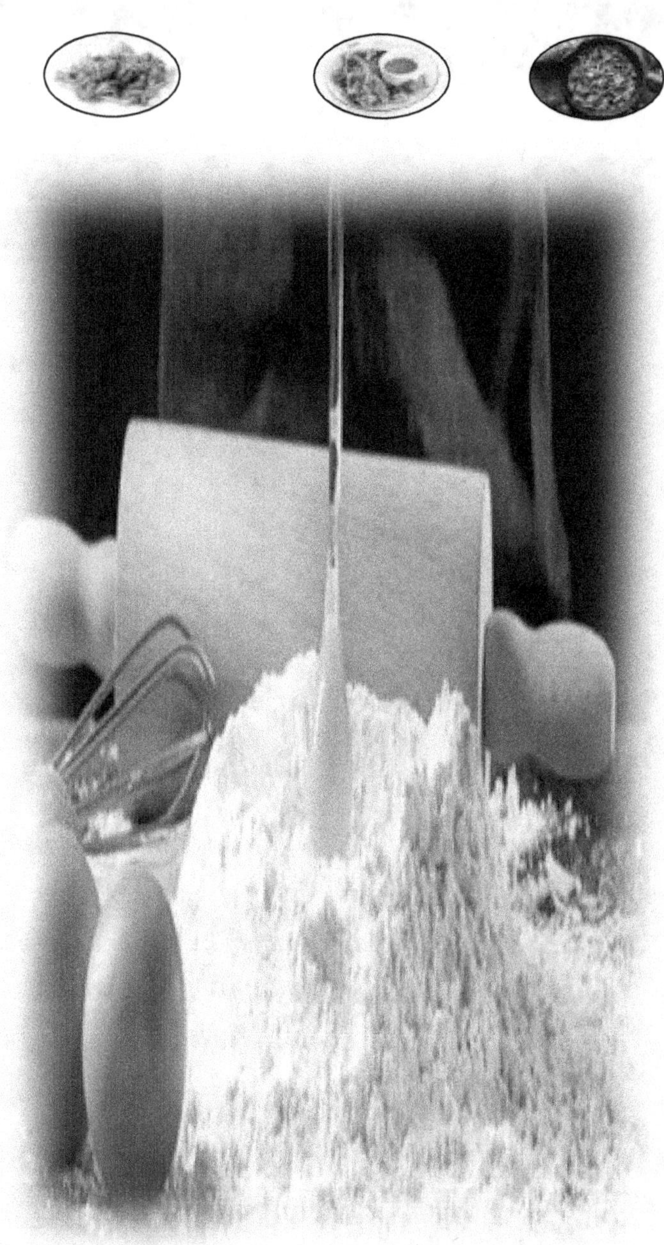

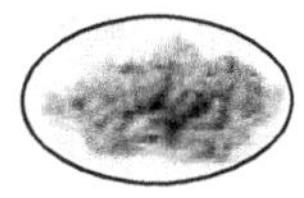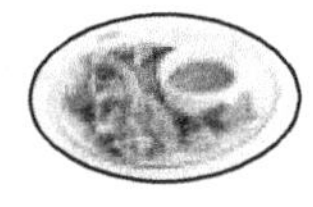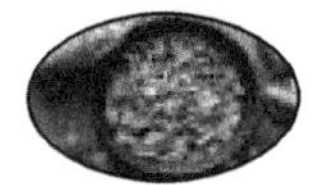

TABLE OF CONTENT–

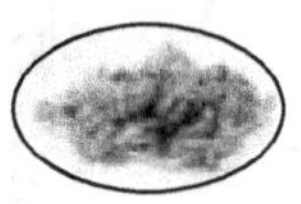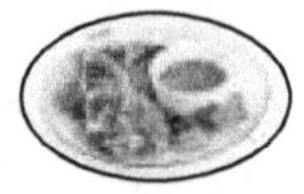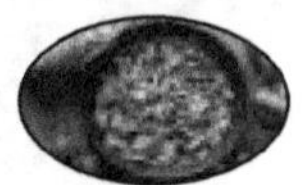

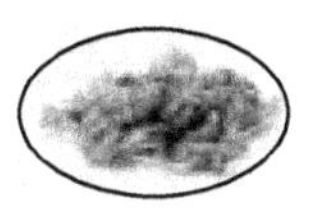 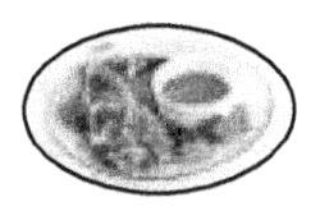 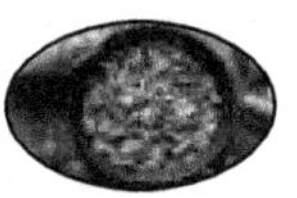

Diet

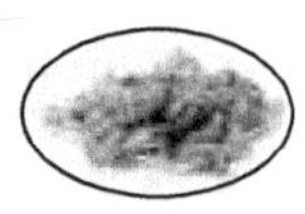 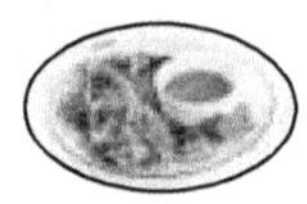 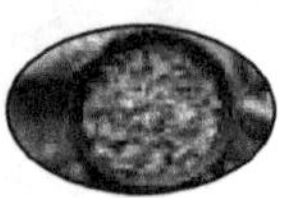

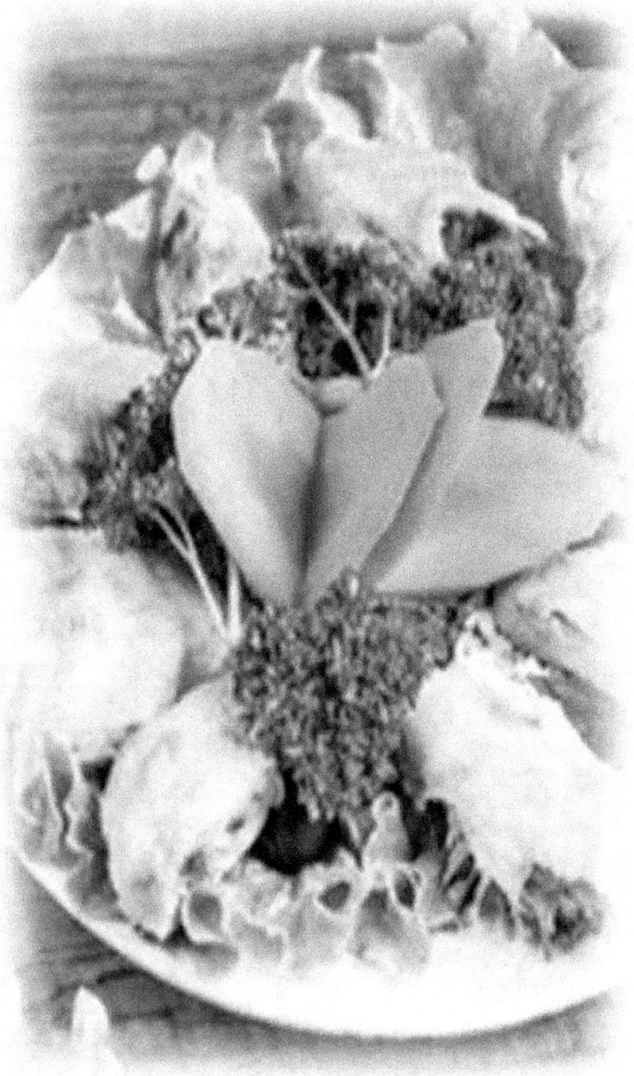

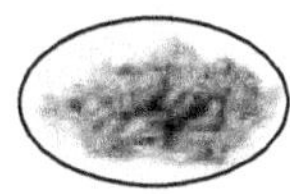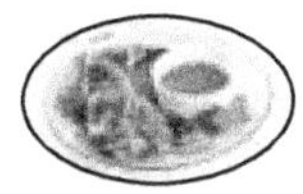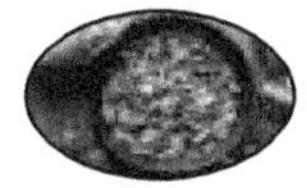

Anti-inflammatory DISH

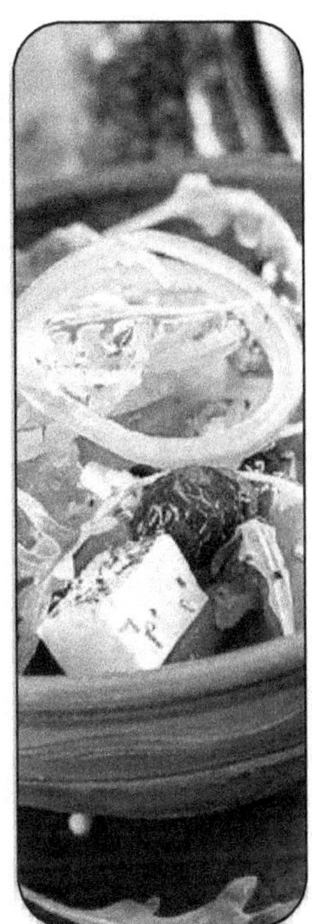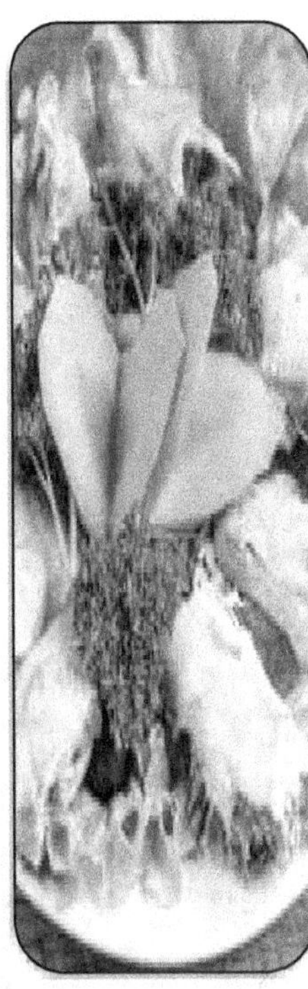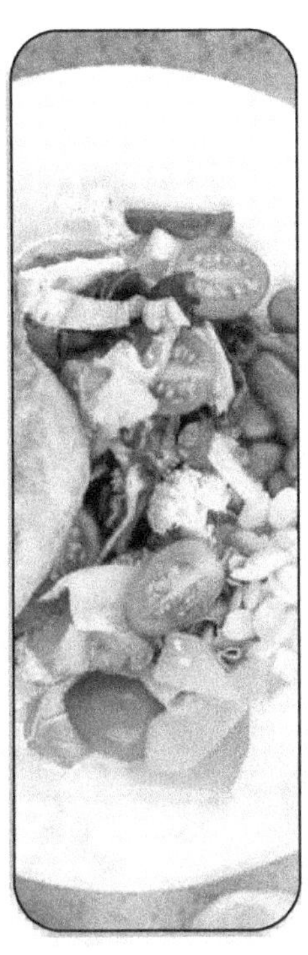

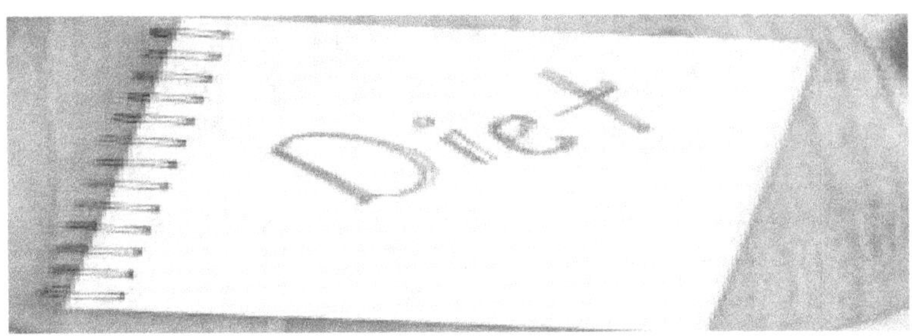

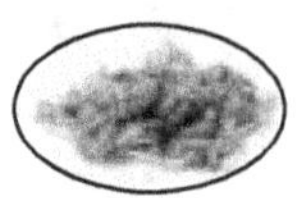 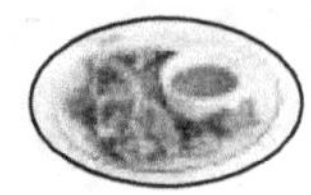 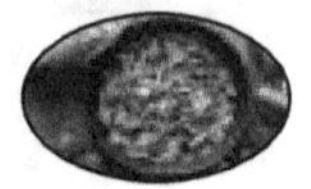

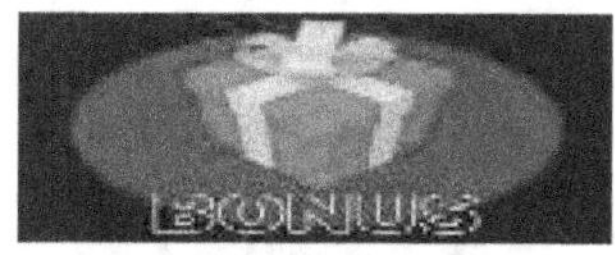

SCAN THE QR CODE TO GET YOUR FREE HOME MADE GREEN SMOOTHIE RECIPE BOOK

BONUS 1

Your 20 days meal planner is attached at the end of the book. Enjoy!

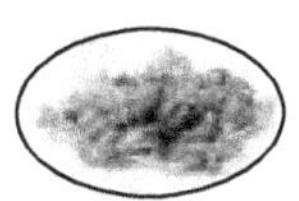 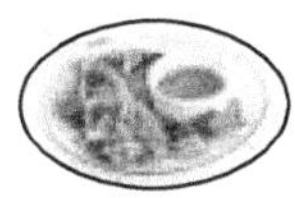 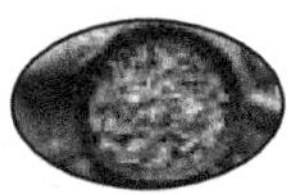

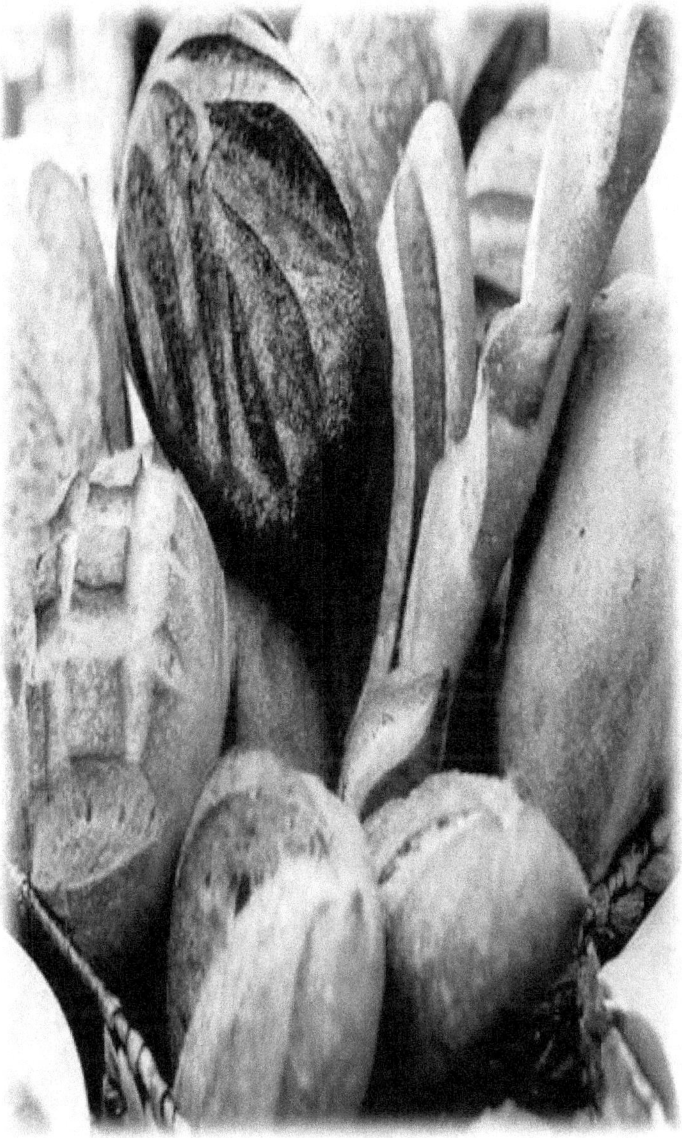

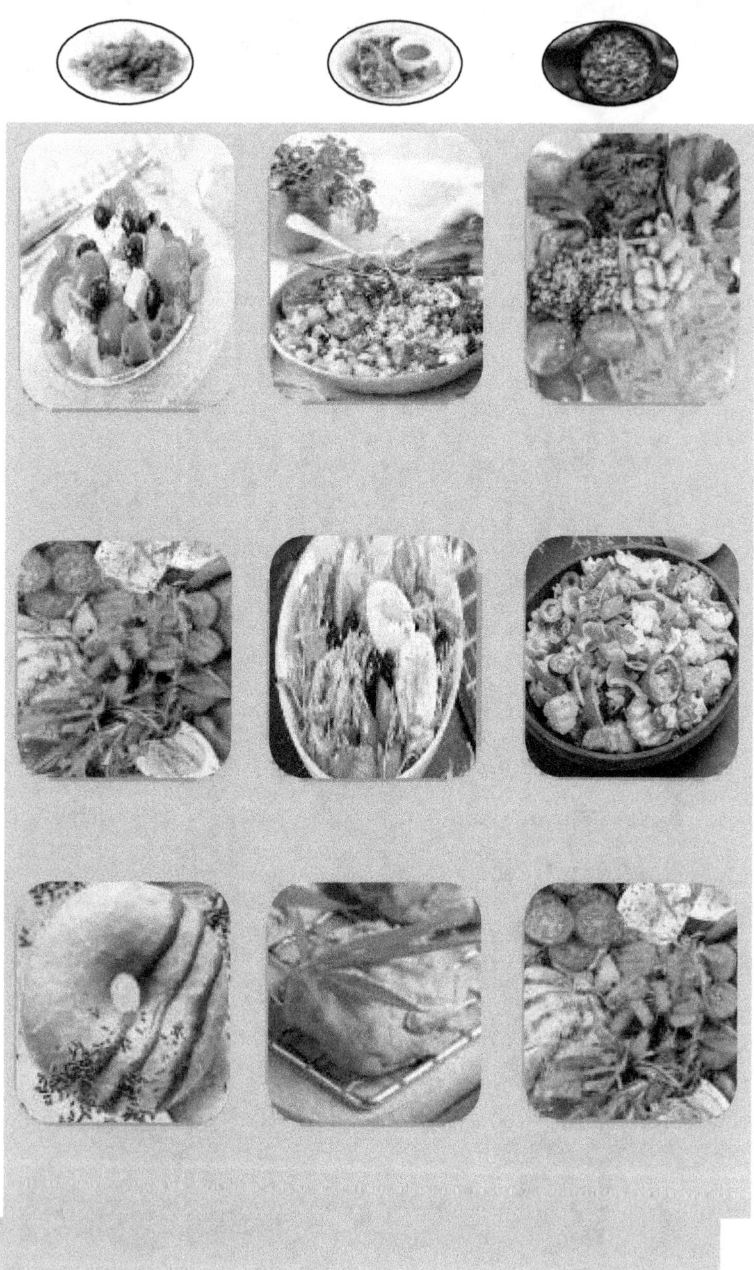

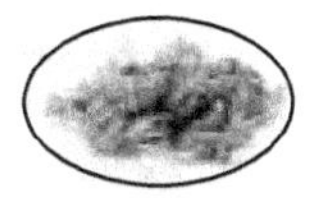 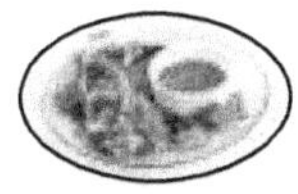 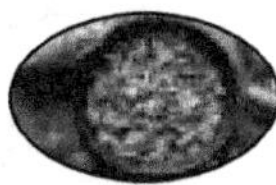

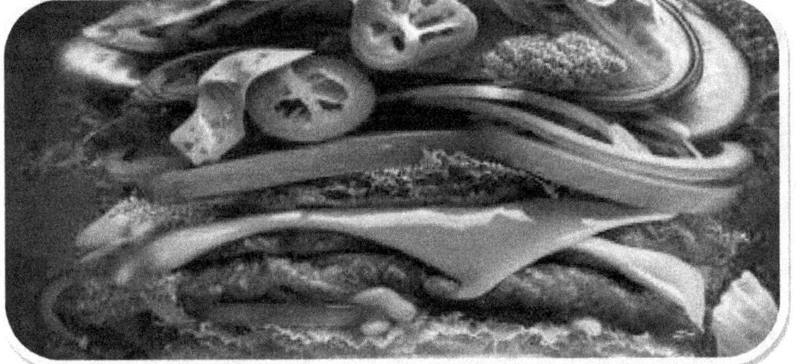

INTRODUCTION–

Once upon a time in a quaint town, the Thompson family found themselves at a crossroads in their health journey. The hustle and bustle of daily life had taken a toll, and the family was seeking a transformative change. It was during these challenging times that they stumbled upon the "28-Day Anti-Inflammatory Diet Book."

Curious and hopeful, the Thompsons decided to embark on this culinary adventure together. Little did they know that this journey would not only revolutionize their approach to food but also strengthen the bonds that held their family together.–

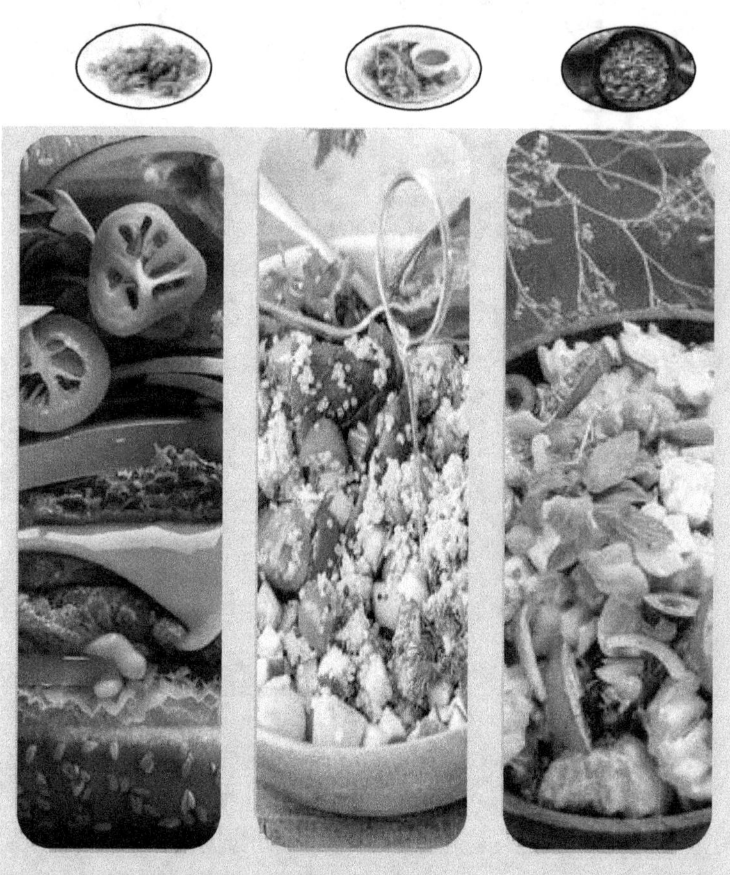

As the days unfolded, the family dove into the vibrant world of turmeric-roasted vegetables, quinoa salads, and innovative smoothie bowls. Each recipe brought with it a burst of flavors and a nourishing touch that resonated with their bodies. The kitchen became a hub of creativity, laughter, and shared moments, as the family discovered the joy of preparing wholesome meals together.

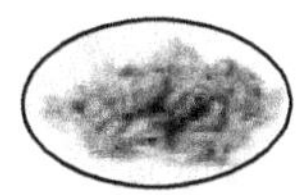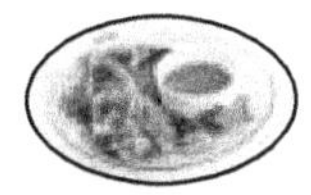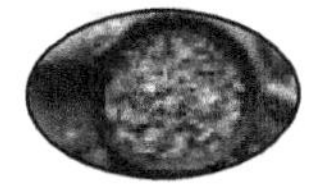

The tangible and intangible benefits began to unfold. Not only did the Thompsons witness a positive shift in their overall well-being, but they also found themselves more connected as a family. The shared experiences of experimenting with new ingredients, exploring diverse flavors, and savoring delicious, healthful meals became the cornerstone of their newfound vitality.

The children, once hesitant about veggies, transformed into little sous-chefs, excitedly chopping and mixing ingredients. The aroma of fresh herbs and spices wafted through the Thompson household, creating an atmosphere that radiated warmth and togetherness.

Through this culinary exploration, the family not only embraced the anti-inflammatory principles but also adopted a holistic approach to health. It became more than just a diet; it became a lifestyle—one that nourished their bodies, minds, and souls.

As the 28-day challenge unfolded, the Thompsons emerged as a healthier, happier, and more harmonious family. The shared meals, the joy of discovering new flavors, and the positive impact on their well-being became the catalyst for a life-altering transformation.

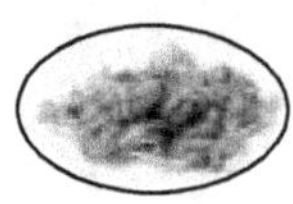 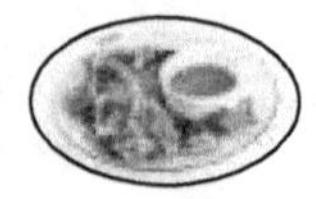 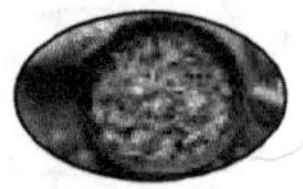

So, dear reader, as you embark on this journey through the pages of the "28-Day Anti-Inflammatory Diet Book," may you find not just recipes but a pathway to a healthier, more connected, and vibrant life—one that the Thompson family discovered, one delicious recipe at a time.

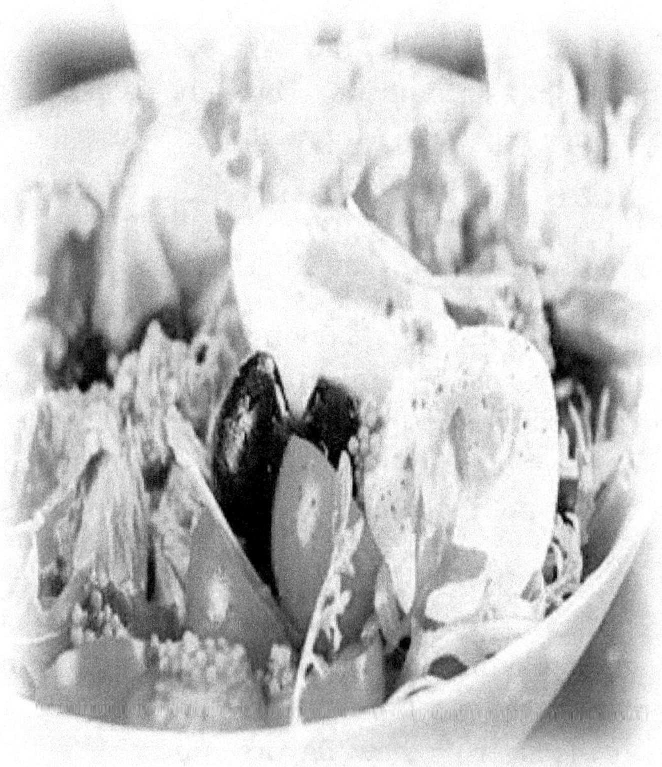

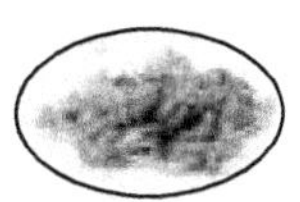 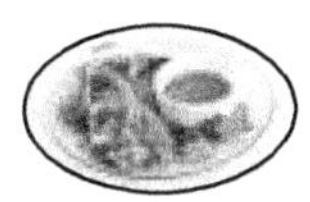 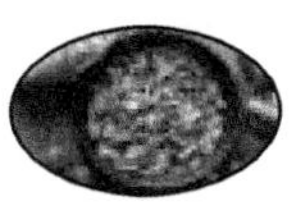

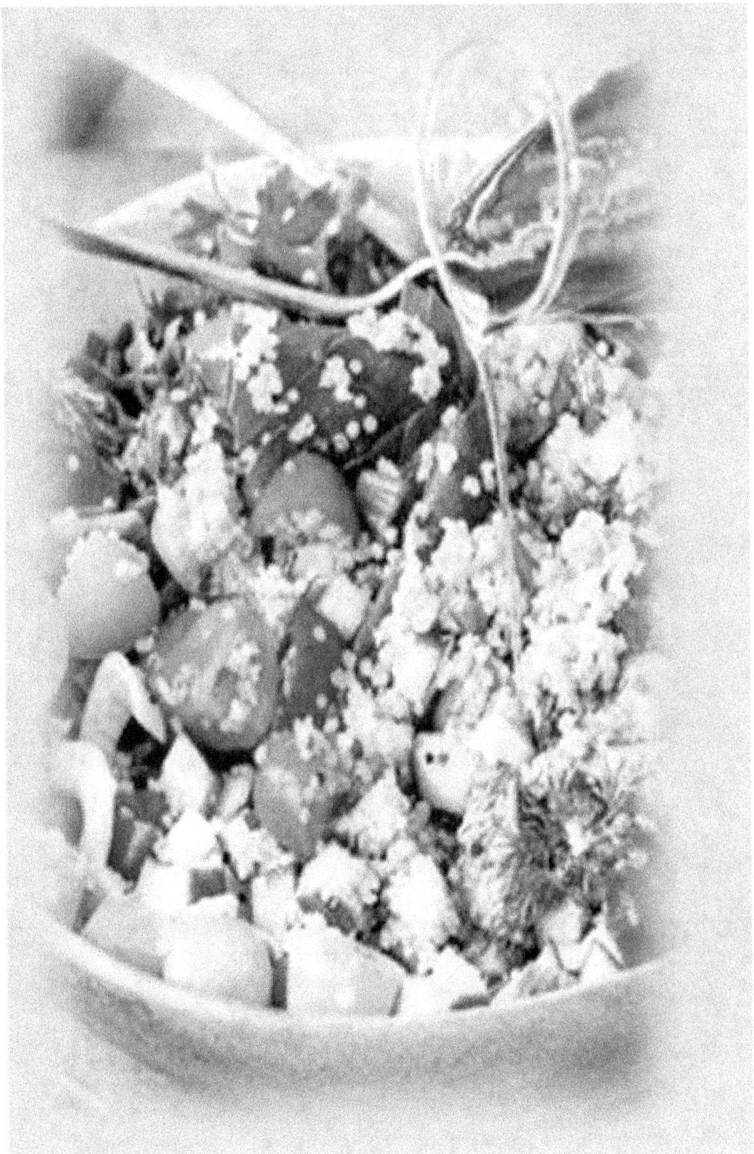

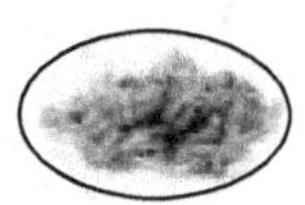 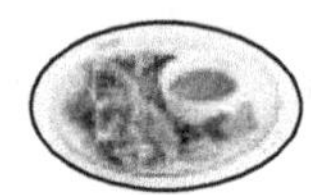 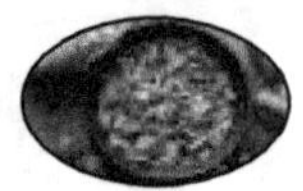

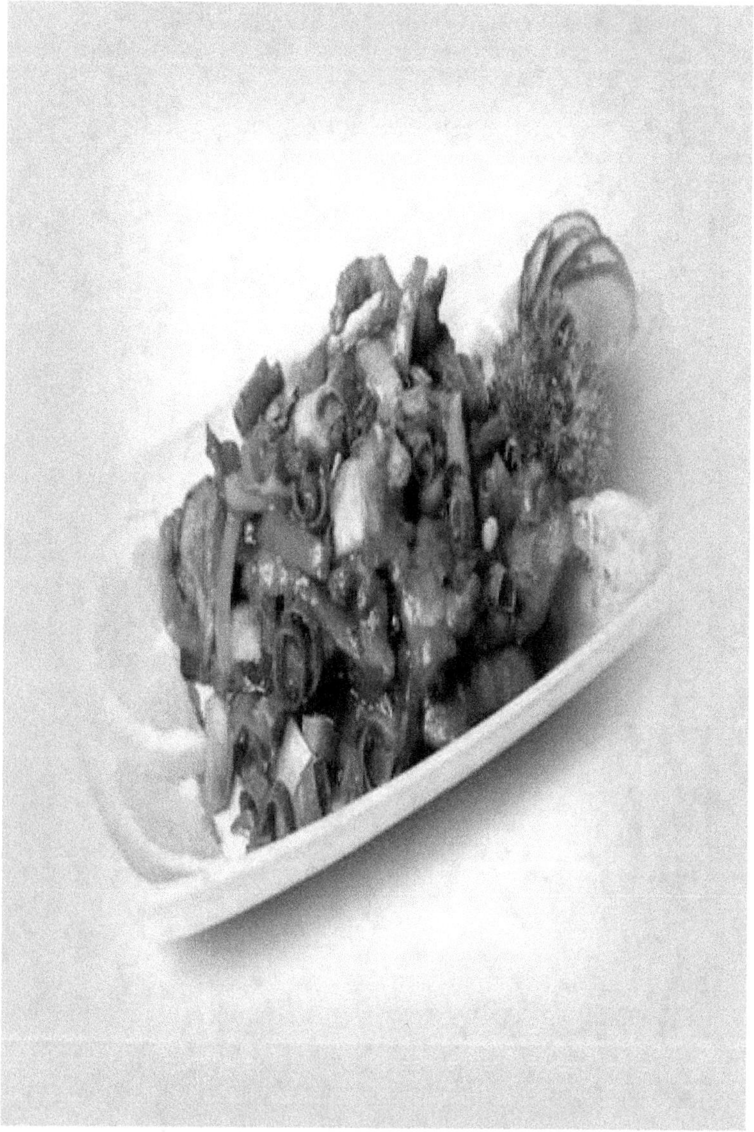

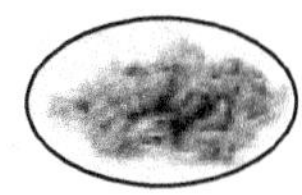 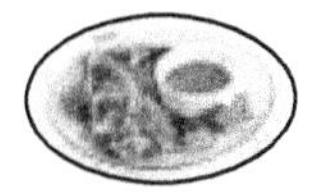 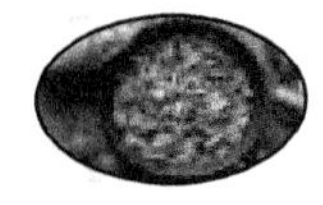

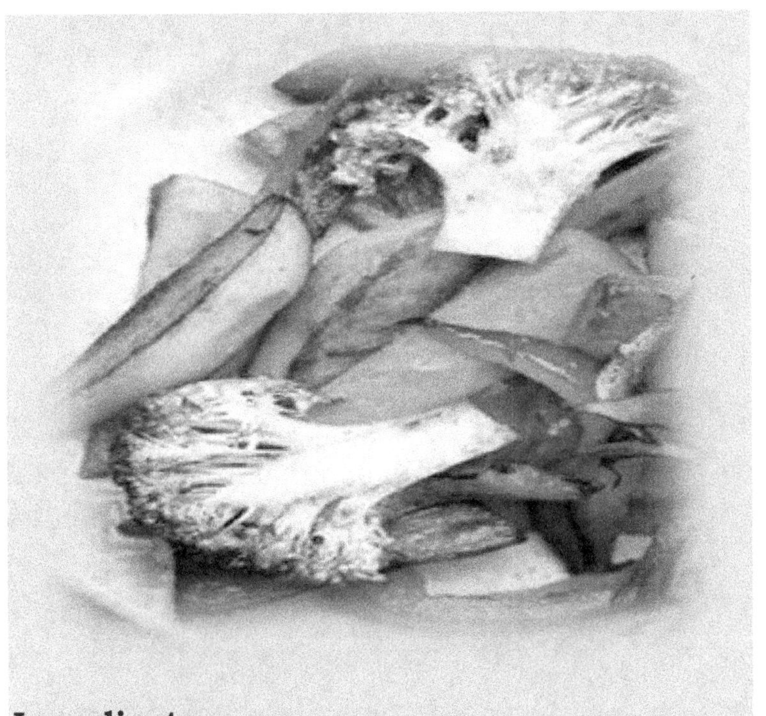

Ingredients:

- 2 cups broccoli florets

- 2 cups cauliflower florets

- 1 bell pepper, sliced

- 1 zucchini, sliced

- 2 tablespoons olive oil

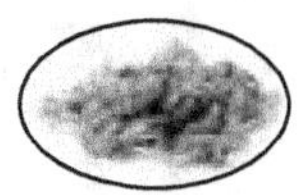 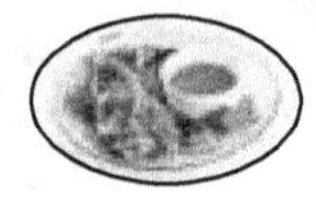 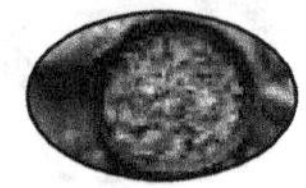

- 1 teaspoon turmeric powder

- 1/2 teaspoon garlic powder

- Salt and pepper to taste

Instructions:

1. Preheat oven to 400°F (200°C).

2. In a large bowl, toss broccoli, cauliflower, bell pepper, and zucchini with olive oil.

3. Sprinkle turmeric and garlic powder evenly over vegetables; toss to coat.

4. Spread vegetables on a baking sheet and roast for 20-25 minutes, or until tender.

5. Season with salt and pepper before serving.

2. Quinoa Salad with Avocado and Almonds

Ingredients:

- 1 cup quinoa, cooked

- 1 avocado, diced

- 1/4 cup sliced almonds

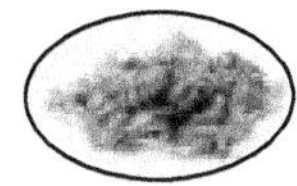 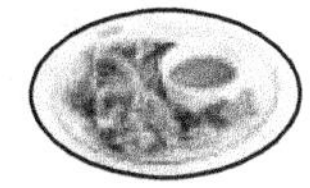 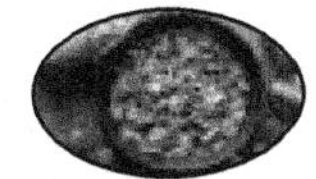

- 2 tablespoons olive oil

- 1 tablespoon lemon juice

- 1 teaspoon honey

- Salt and pepper to taste

- Fresh cilantro for garnish

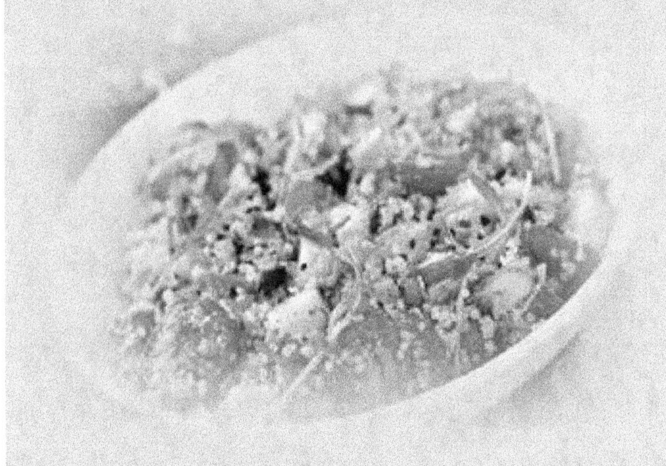

Instructions:

1. In a bowl, combine cooked quinoa, diced avocado, and sliced almonds.

2. In a small bowl, whisk together olive oil, lemon juice, honey, salt, and pepper.

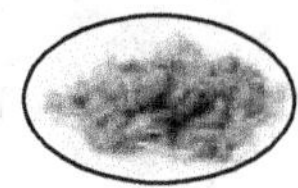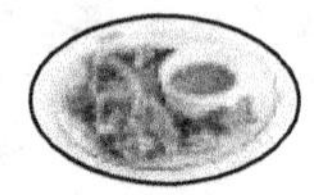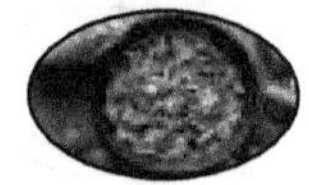

3. After adding the dressing to the quinoa mixture, toss to blend.

4. Garnish with fresh cilantro before serving.

3. Salmon and Asparagus Foil Packets

Ingredients:

- 2 salmon fillets

- 1 bunch asparagus, trimmed

- 2 tablespoons olive oil

- 1 teaspoon dried dill

- 1/2 teaspoon garlic powder

- Lemon slices

- Salt and pepper to taste

Instructions:

1. Preheat the oven to 375°F (190°C).

2. Place each salmon fillet on a piece of foil; surround with asparagus.

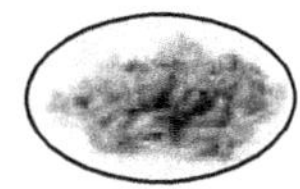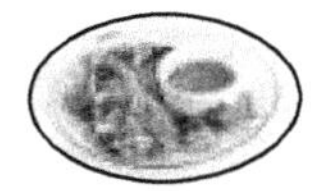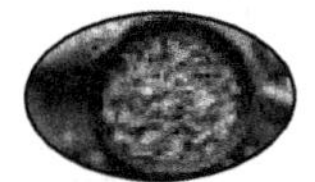

3. Drizzle olive oil over salmon and asparagus; sprinkle with dried dill and garlic powder.

4. Add lemon slices on top and season with salt and pepper.

5. Seal the foil packets and bake for 20-25 minutes.

4. Spinach and Berry Smoothie

Ingredients:

- 2 cups fresh spinach

- One cup of mixed berries, comprising blueberries, raspberries, and strawberries

- 1 banana

- 1 cup almond milk

- 1 tablespoon chia seeds

- Ice cubes (optional)–

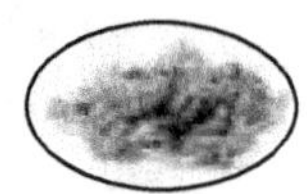 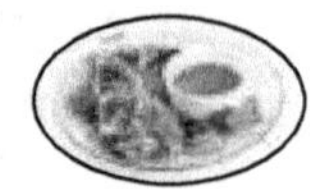 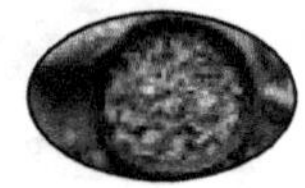

Instructions:

1. Blend spinach, mixed berries, banana, and almond milk until smooth.

2. Add chia seeds and blend for an additional 10 seconds.

3. Add ice cubes if desired and blend until well combined.

4. Pour into a glass and enjoy this refreshing anti-inflammatory smoothie.

5. Chickpea and Vegetable Stir-Fry

Ingredients:

- 1 can chickpeas, drained and rinsed

- Two cups of mixed veggies, such as bell peppers, broccoli, and snap peas

- 2 tablespoons olive oil

- 1 tablespoon soy sauce

- 1 teaspoon ginger, minced

- 1 teaspoon turmeric powder

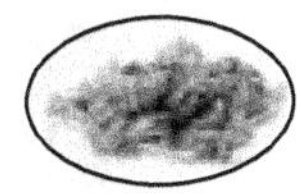 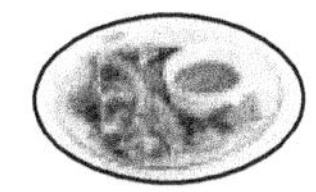 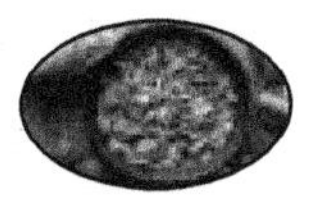

- Brown rice (optional, for serving)

Instructions:

1. Heat olive oil in a pan; add chickpeas and mixed vegetables.

2. Stir in soy sauce, ginger, and turmeric powder; cook until vegetables are tender.

3. Serve over brown rice if desired.

6. Sweet Potato and Kale Hash

Ingredients:

- 2 sweet potatoes, diced

- 2 cups kale, chopped

- 1 onion, finely chopped

- 2 tablespoons coconut oil

- 1 teaspoon cumin

- 1/2 teaspoon smoked paprika

- Salt and pepper to taste–

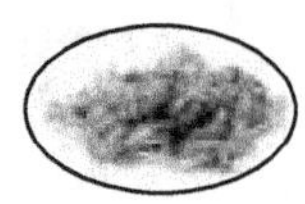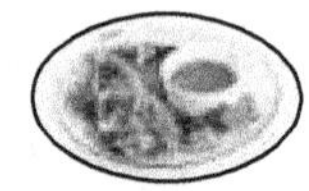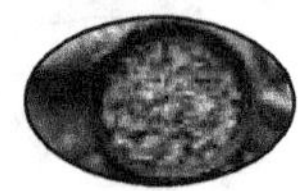

Instructions:

1. In a skillet, heat coconut oil over medium heat; add diced sweet potatoes and onion.

2. Cook until sweet potatoes are golden brown and tender.

3. Add chopped kale, cumin, smoked paprika, salt, and pepper; stir until kale is wilted.

7. Lemon Garlic Chicken Skewers

Ingredients:

- 2 chicken breasts, cut into cubes

- 2 lemons, juiced

- 3 cloves garlic, minced

- 2 tablespoons olive oil

- 1 teaspoon dried oregano

- Salt and pepper to taste–

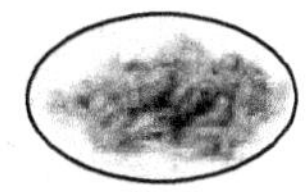 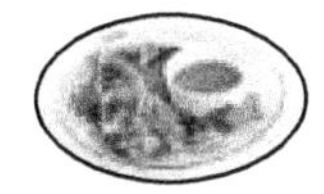 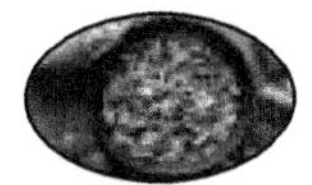

Instructions:

1. In a bowl, combine lemon juice, minced garlic, olive oil, oregano, salt, and pepper.

2. Add chicken cubes to the marinade, coating evenly.

3. Thread chicken onto skewers and grill for 10-12 minutes, turning occasionally.

8. Cauliflower Rice Stir-Fry

Ingredients:

- 1 head cauliflower, grated

- 1 cup mixed vegetables (carrots, peas, corn)

- 2 eggs, beaten

- 3 tablespoons coconut aminos

- 1 tablespoon sesame oil

- Green onions for garnish–

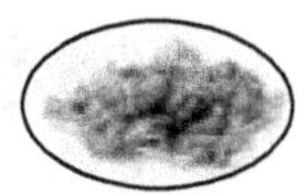 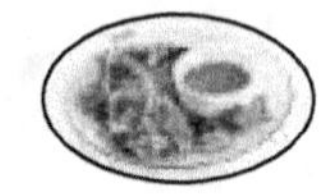 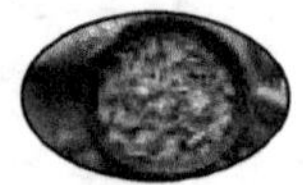

Instructions:

1. In a pan, sauté cauliflower rice and mixed vegetables until tender.

2. Push the rice mixture to the side and pour beaten eggs into the pan.

3. Scramble the eggs and mix with the rice.

4. Stir in coconut aminos and sesame oil; garnish with green onions.

9. Mango Avocado Salsa

Ingredients:

- 1 ripe mango, diced

- 1 avocado, diced

- 1/2 red onion, finely chopped

- 1 jalapeño, seeded and minced

- Fresh cilantro, chopped

- Lime juice

- Salt and pepper to taste–

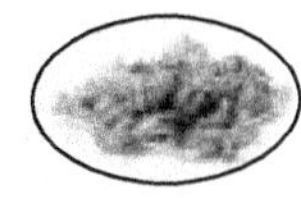 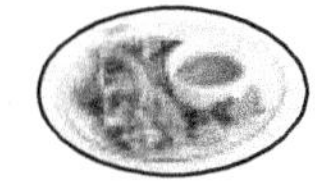 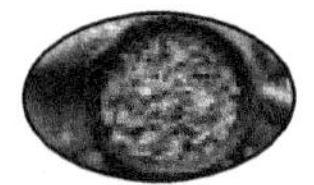

Instructions:

1. In a bowl, combine diced mango, avocado, red onion, jalapeño, and cilantro.

2. Drizzle lime juice over the mixture and season with salt and pepper.

3. Gently toss the ingredients together and refrigerate before serving.

10. Broccoli and Lentil Soup

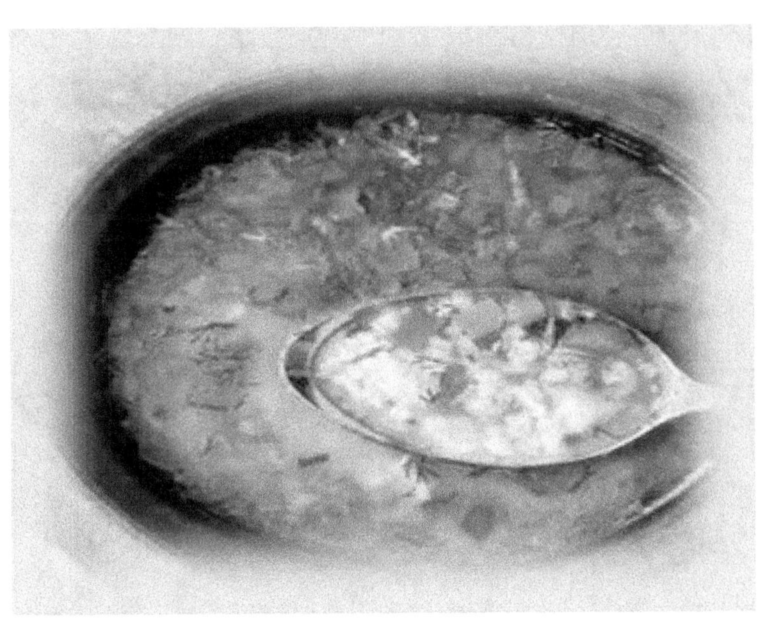

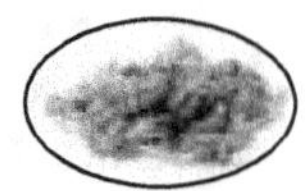 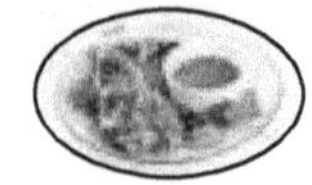 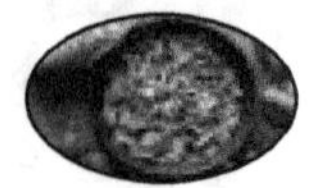

Ingredients:

- 2 cups broccoli florets

- 1 cup dried lentils, rinsed

- 1 onion, diced

- 2 cloves garlic, minced

- 4 cups vegetable broth

- 1 teaspoon cumin

- 1/2 teaspoon turmeric

- Salt and pepper to taste

Instructions:

1. In a pot, sauté onion and garlic until softened.

2. Add broccoli, lentils, vegetable broth, cumin, turmeric, salt, and pepper.

3. Bring to a boil, then reduce heat and simmer until lentils are cooked and broccoli is tender.–

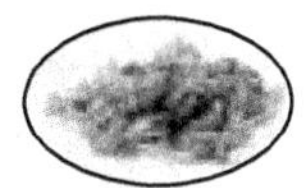 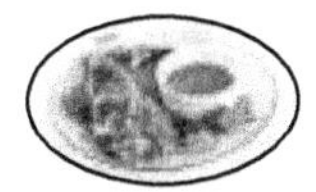 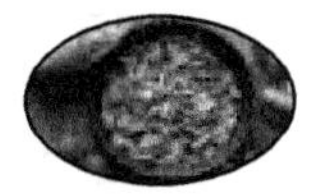

Ingredients:

- 2 cod fillets
- 1 lemon, sliced
- 2 tablespoons olive oil
- 1 teaspoon dried thyme
- 1/2 teaspoon onion powder
- Salt and pepper to taste
- Fresh parsley for garnish

Instructions:

1. Preheat the oven to 375°F (190°C).
2. Place cod fillets on a baking dish; drizzle with olive oil.
3. Season with dried thyme, onion powder, salt, and pepper.
4. Arrange lemon slices on top of the cod.
5. Bake for 15-20 minutes or until the fish flakes easily.

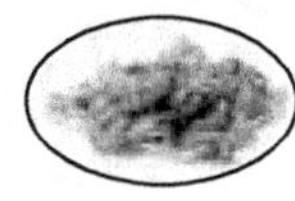 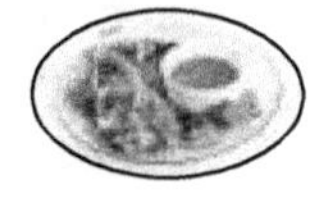 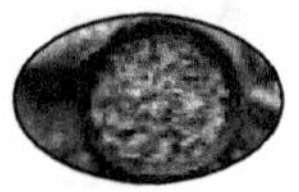

6. Garnish with fresh parsley before serving.

12. Spaghetti Squash with Pesto and Cherry Tomatoes

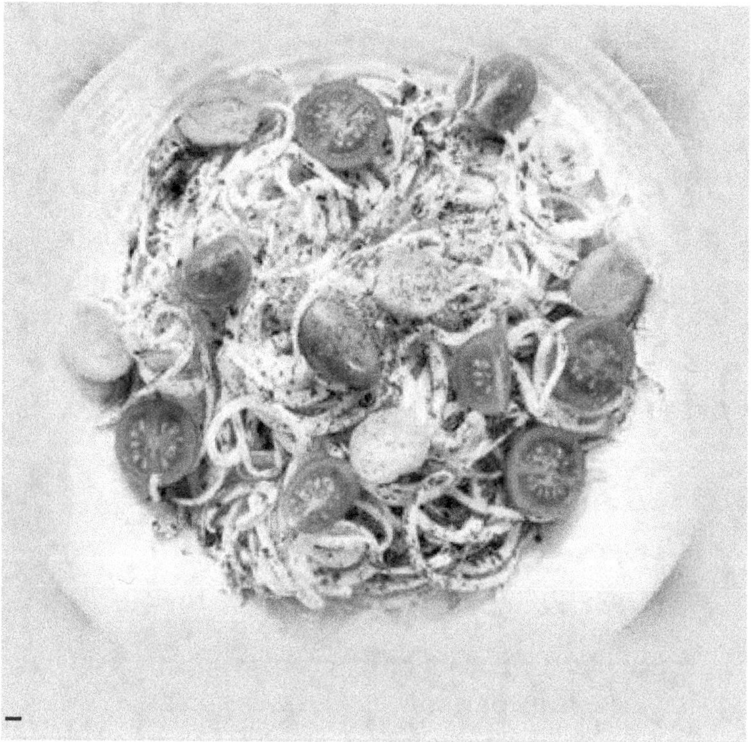

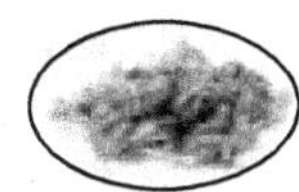 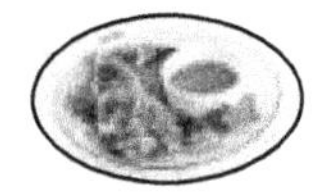 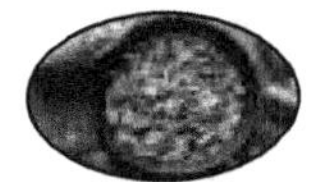

Ingredients:

- 1 spaghetti squash, halved and seeded

- 1 cup cherry tomatoes, halved

- 1/4 cup pine nuts

- 1/2 cup fresh basil leaves

- 1/4 cup grated Parmesan cheese

- 2 cloves garlic

- 3 tablespoons olive oil

- Salt and pepper to taste

Instructions:

1. Roast spaghetti squash in the oven at 400°F (200°C) for 40-45 minutes.

2. In a blender, combine basil, pine nuts, Parmesan, garlic, olive oil, salt, and pepper.

3. Scrape the cooked spaghetti squash with a fork to create "noodles."

4. Toss squash noodles with pesto and cherry tomatoes.–

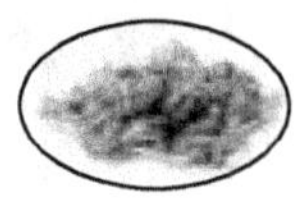 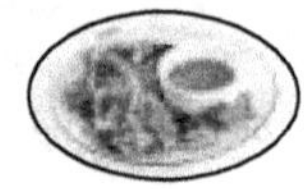 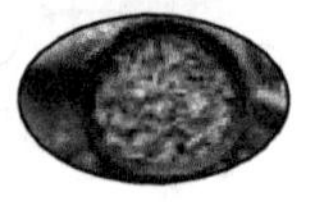

Ingredients:

- 1 cup mixed berries (blueberries, strawberries)

- 1 banana

- 1 cup spinach

- 1/2 cup brewed green tea, cooled

- 2 tablespoons chia seeds

- Granola for topping (optional)

Instructions:

1. Blend mixed berries, banana, spinach, and green tea until smooth.

2. Pour into a bowl and sprinkle chia seeds on top.

3. Optionally, add granola for crunch.

4. Enjoy this antioxidant-rich smoothie bowl!–

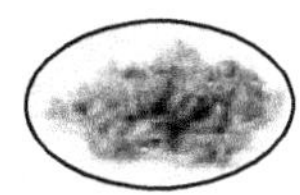 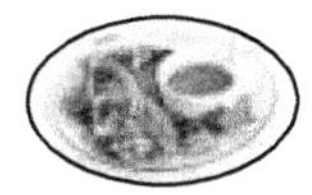 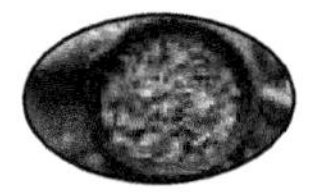

Ingredients:

- 2 cucumbers, thinly sliced

- 1 avocado, diced

- 1/4 cup red onion, thinly sliced

- 2 tablespoons olive oil

- 1 tablespoon apple cider vinegar

- Fresh dill for garnish

- Salt and pepper to taste

Instructions:

1. In a bowl, combine cucumber, avocado, and red onion.

2. Whisk together olive oil, apple cider vinegar, salt, and pepper.

3. Pour the dressing over the salad and give it a little stir.

4. Garnish with fresh dill before serving.–

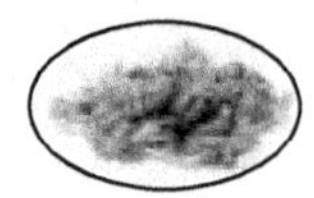 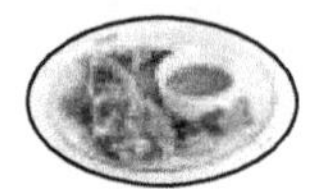 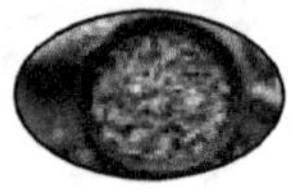

Ingredients:

- 3 eggs, beaten

- 1 cup mushrooms, sliced

- 1 cup fresh spinach leaves

- 1/4 cup feta cheese, crumbled

- 1 tablespoon olive oil

- Salt and pepper to taste

Instructions:

1. In a pan, sauté mushrooms and spinach in olive oil until wilted.

2. Pour beaten eggs over the vegetables; cook until the edges set.

3. Sprinkle crumbled feta over one half of the omelette.

4. Fold the omelette in half and cook until the cheese melts.–

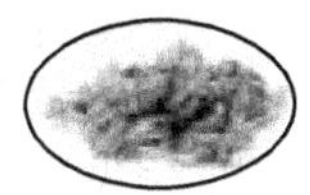 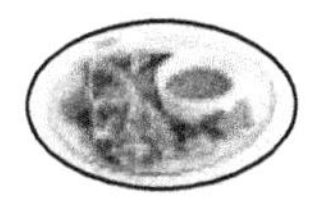 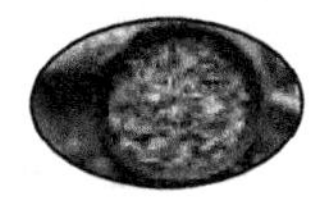

Ingredients:

- 2 sweet potatoes, cut into fries

- 2 tablespoons olive oil

- 1 teaspoon paprika

- 1/2 teaspoon cayenne pepper

- 1/2 teaspoon cinnamon

- Salt and pepper to taste

Instructions:

1. Preheat the oven to 425°F (220°C).

2. Toss sweet potato fries with olive oil, paprika, cayenne pepper, cinnamon, salt, and pepper.

3. Spread fries in a single layer on a baking sheet.

4. Bake for 20-25 minutes, flipping halfway through.–

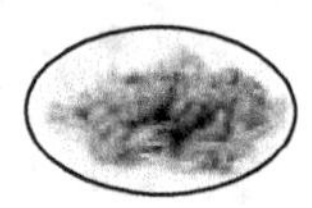 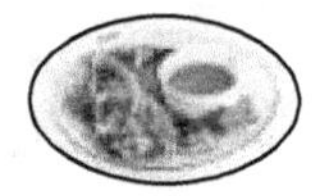 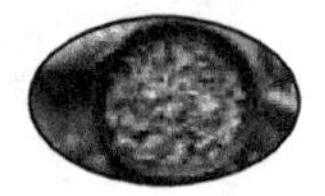

Ingredients:

- 1 can tuna, drained
- 1 can white beans, rinsed and drained
- 1 cucumber, diced
- 1/4 cup red bell pepper, chopped
- 2 tablespoons olive oil
- 1 tablespoon balsamic vinegar
- Fresh parsley for garnish
- Salt and pepper to taste

Instructions:

1. In a bowl, combine tuna, white beans, cucumber, and red bell pepper.

2. Whisk together olive oil, balsamic vinegar, salt, and pepper.

3. After adding the dressing, gently mix the salad.

4. Garnish with fresh parsley before serving.

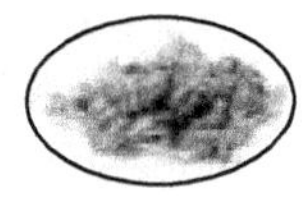 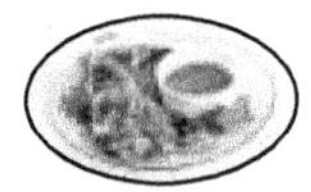 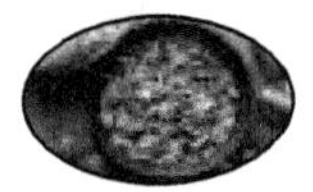

Ingredients:

- 1/2 cup rolled oats
- 1/2 cup almond milk
- 1/4 cup blueberries
- 1 tablespoon almond butter
- 1 teaspoon honey
- Sliced almonds for topping

Instructions:

1. In a jar, combine rolled oats, almond milk, blueberries, almond butter, and honey.

2. Stir well, cover, and refrigerate overnight.

3. In the morning, top with sliced almonds before enjoying.–

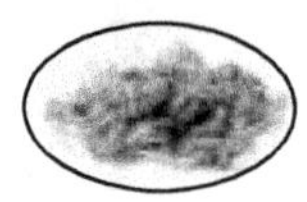 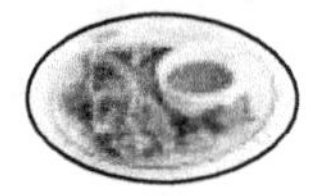 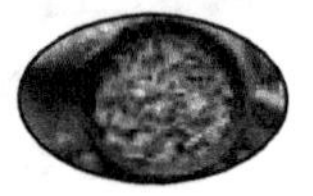

Ingredients:

- 2 chicken breasts, cut into cubes
- 1 zucchini, sliced
- 1 red onion, cut into chunks
- 1 bell pepper, cut into chunks
- 3 tablespoons olive oil
- 1 teaspoon dried oregano
- 1/2 teaspoon garlic powder
- Lemon wedges for serving
- Salt and pepper to taste

Instructions:

1. In a bowl, combine olive oil, dried oregano, garlic powder, salt, and pepper.

2. Thread chicken and vegetables onto skewers, alternating.

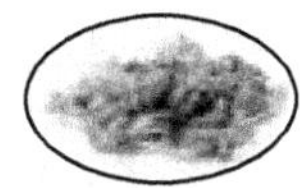 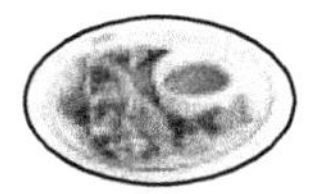 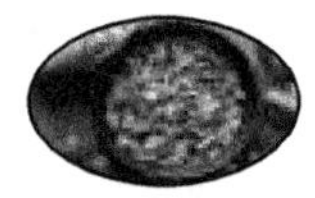

3. Brush skewers with the Mediterranean marinade.

4. Grill for 10-12 minutes, turning occasionally.

5. Present with slices of lemon..

20. Pumpkin and Ginger Soup

Ingredients:

- 2 cups pumpkin, diced

- 1 onion, chopped

- 2 cloves garlic, minced

- 1 tablespoon fresh ginger, grated

- 4 cups vegetable broth

- 1/2 teaspoon ground cinnamon

- 1/4 teaspoon nutmeg

- Coconut milk for garnish

- Salt and pepper to taste–

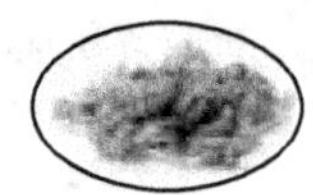 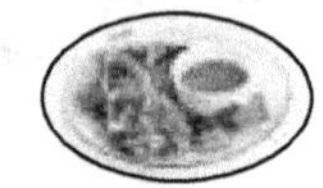 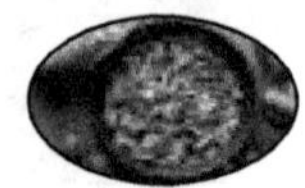

Instructions:

1. In a pot, sauté onion, garlic, and ginger until fragrant.

2. Add diced pumpkin, vegetable broth, ground cinnamon, nutmeg, salt, and pepper.

3. Simmer until the pumpkin is tender.

4. Blend until smooth and serve with a drizzle of coconut milk.

21. Lentil and Vegetable Curry

Ingredients:

- 1 cup dried lentils, rinsed

- Two cups of mixed veggies (cauliflower, peas, carrots)

- 1 onion, finely chopped

- 2 cloves garlic, minced

- 1 can coconut milk

- 2 tablespoons curry powder

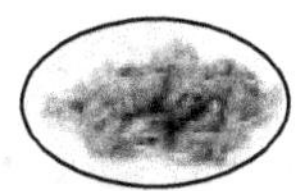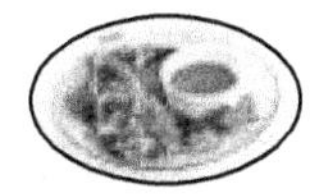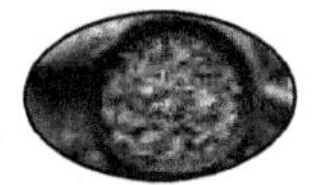

- 1 teaspoon turmeric

- Fresh cilantro for garnish

- Salt and pepper to taste

Instructions:

1. Cook lentils according to package instructions.

2. In a pan, sauté onion and garlic until softened.

3. Add mixed vegetables, curry powder, turmeric, salt, and pepper; cook until vegetables are tender.

4. Stir in cooked lentils and coconut milk; simmer for 10 minutes.

5. Garnish with fresh cilantro before serving.

22. Brussels Sprouts and Pomegranate Salad

Ingredients:

- 2 cups Brussels sprouts, shredded

- 1/2 cup pomegranate arils

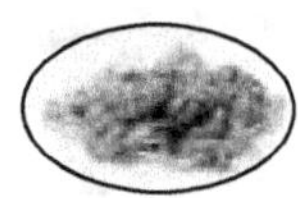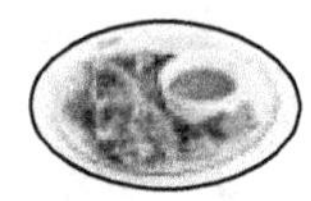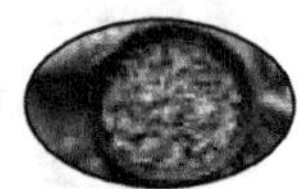

- 1/4 cup feta cheese, crumbled

- 2 tablespoons balsamic vinaigrette

- 1 tablespoon olive oil

- 1 tablespoon honey

- Salt and pepper to taste

Instructions:

1. In a bowl, combine shredded Brussels sprouts, pomegranate arils, and feta cheese.

2. Whisk together balsamic vinaigrette, olive oil, honey, salt, and pepper.

3. Pour the dressing over the salad and give it a little stir.

23. Cabbage and Apple Slaw

Ingredients:

- 1/2 head green cabbage, thinly sliced

- 2 apples, julienned

- 1/4 cup Greek yogurt

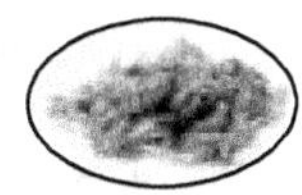 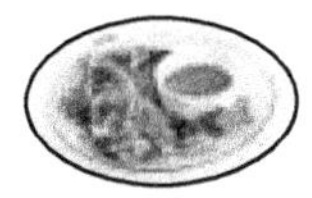 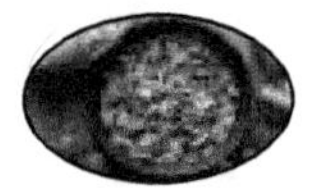

- 1 tablespoon Dijon mustard

- 1 tablespoon apple cider vinegar

- 1 teaspoon honey

- Chopped walnuts for garnish

- Salt and pepper to taste

Instructions:

1. In a bowl, combine sliced cabbage and julienned apples.

2. In a separate bowl, whisk together Greek yogurt, Dijon mustard, apple cider vinegar, honey, salt, and pepper.

3. Pour the dressing over the cabbage and apple mixture; toss well.

4. Garnish with chopped walnuts before serving.

24. Minty Cucumber Infused Water

Ingredients:

- 1 cucumber, thinly sliced

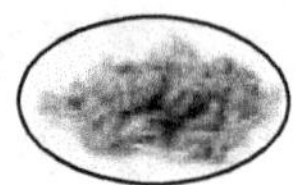 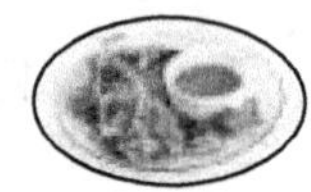 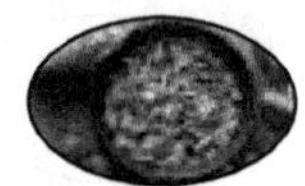

- 1 lemon, thinly sliced

- Fresh mint leaves

- 1.5 liters water

- Ice cubes (optional)

Instructions:

1. In a pitcher, combine cucumber and lemon slices with fresh mint leaves.

2. Add water and let it chill in the refrigerator for at least 2 hours.

3. Serve over ice cubes for a refreshing and hydrating beverage.

25. Grilled Eggplant with Tahini Sauce

Ingredients:

- 2 medium eggplants, sliced

- 3 tablespoons olive oil

- 2 tablespoons tahini

- 1 tablespoon lemon juice

- 1 clove garlic, minced

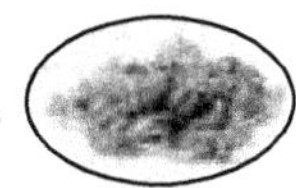 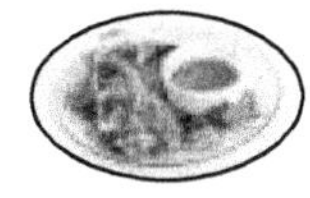 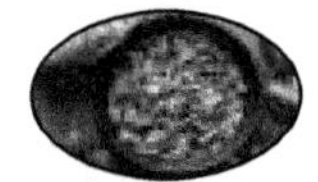

- Fresh parsley for garnish

- Salt and pepper to taste

Instructions:

1. Brush eggplant slices with olive oil and grill for 3-4 minutes on each side.

2. In a bowl, mix tahini, lemon juice, minced garlic, salt, and pepper.

3. Drizzle the tahini sauce over the grilled eggplant.

4. Garnish with fresh parsley before serving.

26. Broccoli and Almond Stir-Fry

Ingredients:

- 2 cups broccoli florets

- 1/2 cup sliced almonds

- 2 tablespoons soy sauce

- 1 tablespoon sesame oil

- 1 teaspoon ginger, minced

- 1 teaspoon honey

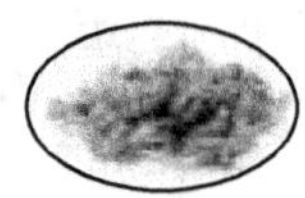 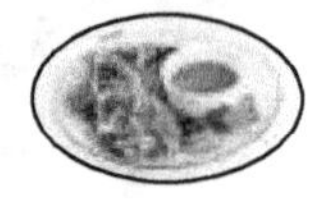 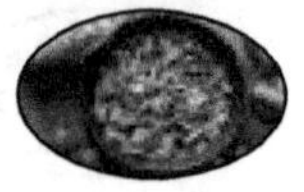

- Brown rice (optional, for serving)

Instructions:

1. Stir-fry broccoli in sesame oil until slightly tender.

2. Add sliced almonds, soy sauce, ginger, and honey; cook until almonds are toasted.

3. Serve over brown rice if desired.

27. Chia Seed Pudding with Berries

Ingredients:

- 1/4 cup chia seeds

- 1 cup almond milk

- 1 tablespoon maple syrup

- 1/2 teaspoon vanilla extract

- Mixed berries for topping–

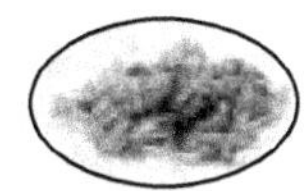 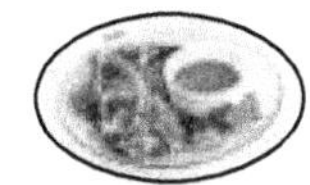 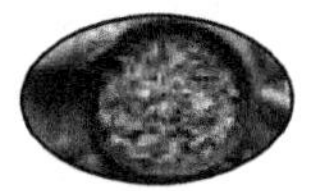

Instructions:

1. In a jar, mix chia seeds, almond milk, maple syrup, and vanilla extract.

2. Stir well, cover, and refrigerate for at least 4 hours or overnight.

3. Top with mixed berries before serving.

28. Cauliflower and Turmeric Soup

Ingredients:

- 1 head cauliflower, chopped

- 1 onion, diced

- 2 cloves garlic, minced

- 4 cups vegetable broth

- 1 teaspoon turmeric

- 1/2 teaspoon cumin

- Coconut milk for garnish

- Salt and pepper to taste

Instructions:

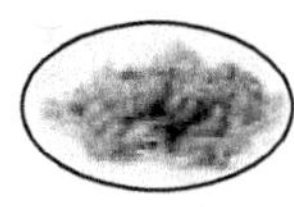 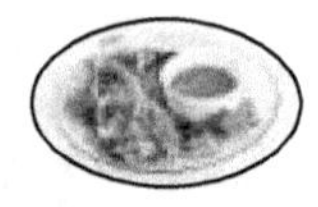 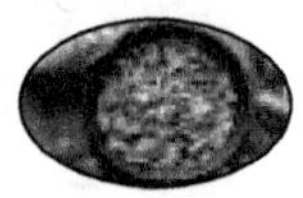

1. Sauté onion and garlic until softened; add chopped cauliflower.

2. Pour in vegetable broth, turmeric, cumin, salt, and pepper; simmer until cauliflower is tender.

3. Blend until smooth and serve with a drizzle of coconut milk.

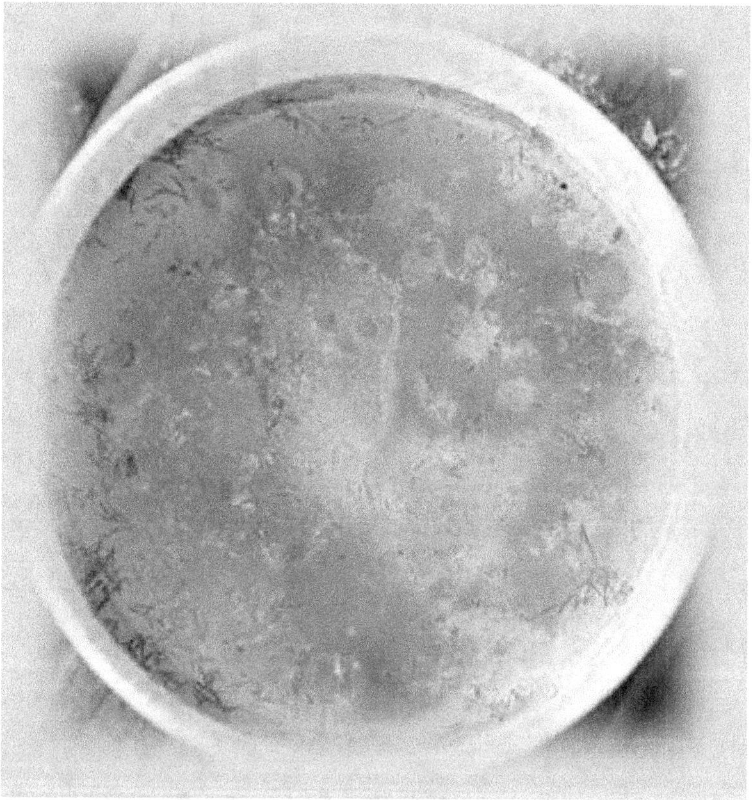

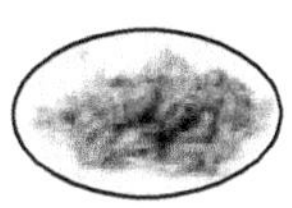 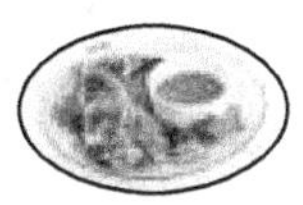 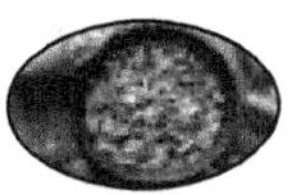

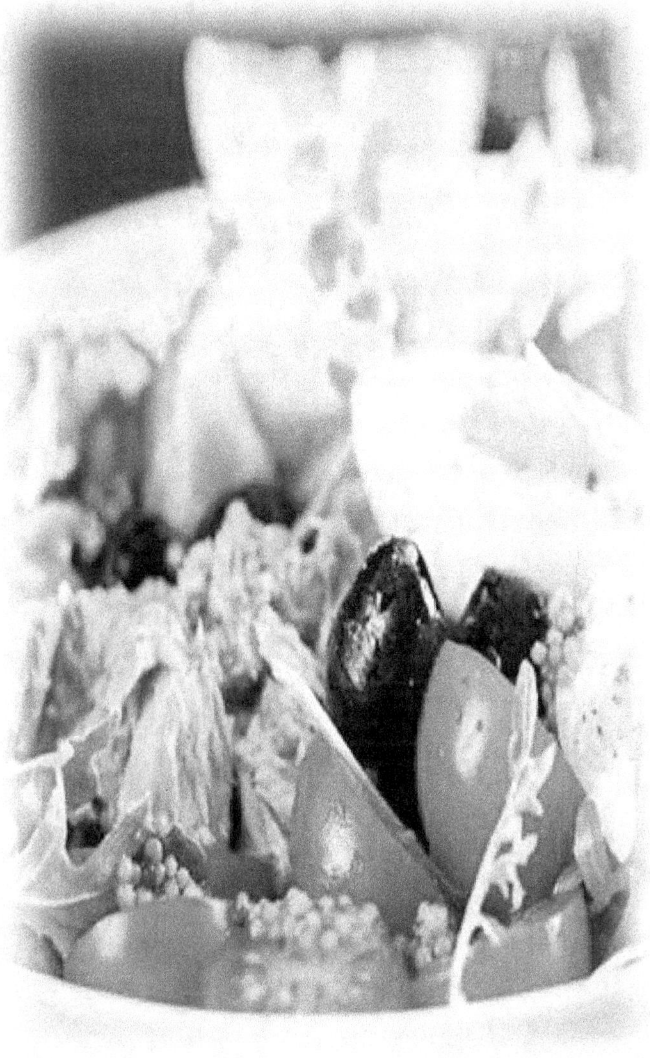

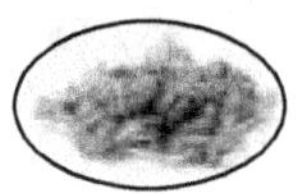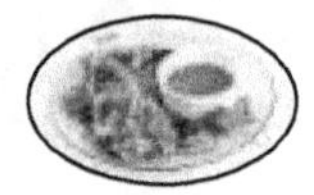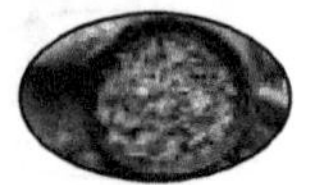

CONCLUSION

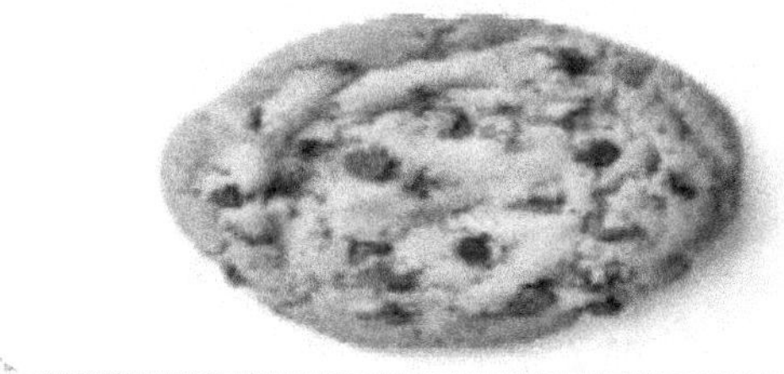

In the closing chapter of our 28-Day Anti-Inflammatory Diet Book, we reflect on the transformative journey that began with a simple desire for better health and culminated in a tapestry of flavorful experiences, strengthened bonds, and newfound vitality.

As you've navigated through the diverse recipes, each carefully crafted to nourish your body and tantalize your taste buds, we hope you've discovered the power that lies within the ingredients you choose. This isn't just a cookbook; it's an invitation to embark on a holistic approach to well-being—one that transcends the boundaries of a mere diet.–

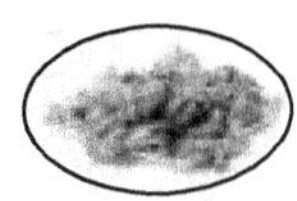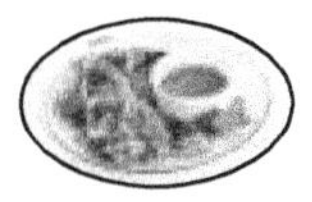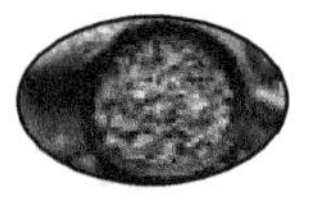

In the footsteps of the Thompson family, may you have felt the joy of creating in the kitchen, relishing the shared moments, and savoring the flavors of healthful living. The journey toward an anti-inflammatory lifestyle is not a solitary one; it's a collective exploration, shared with family, friends, and loved ones.

As you close the pages of this book, let the stories of those who embraced this challenge inspire you. The stories of families who, like you, sought a positive change and found it in the vibrant colors of vegetables, the richness of spices, and the simplicity of mindful eating.

May the knowledge gained during these 28 days become the foundation for a lifelong commitment to your well-being. Remember, it's not about restriction but about embracing the abundance of nourishing choices available to you. The recipes shared here are just the beginning—your canvas to paint a picture of a healthier, more vibrant you.

As you step into this new chapter of your life, may it be filled with continued exploration, joyous kitchen creations, and a radiant sense of well-being.–

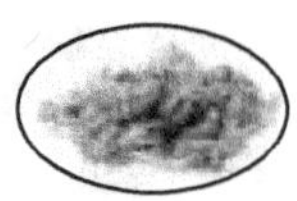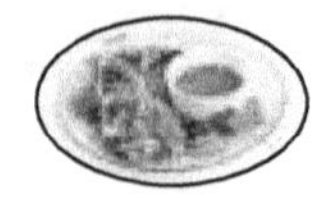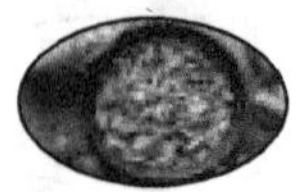

Here's to a future filled with health, happiness, and the endless possibilities that lie within the choices you make for yourself and those you hold dear. Cheers to the next chapter, and may it be as delicious as the recipes you've discovered along the way!

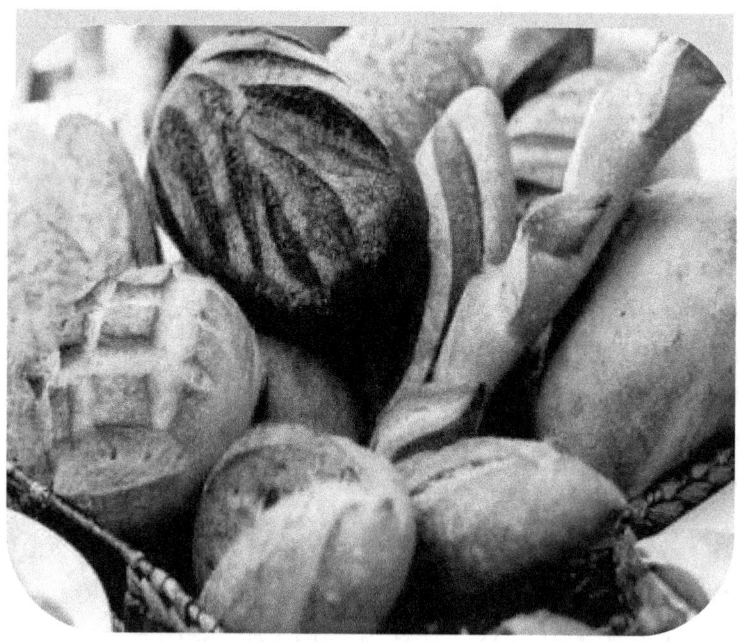

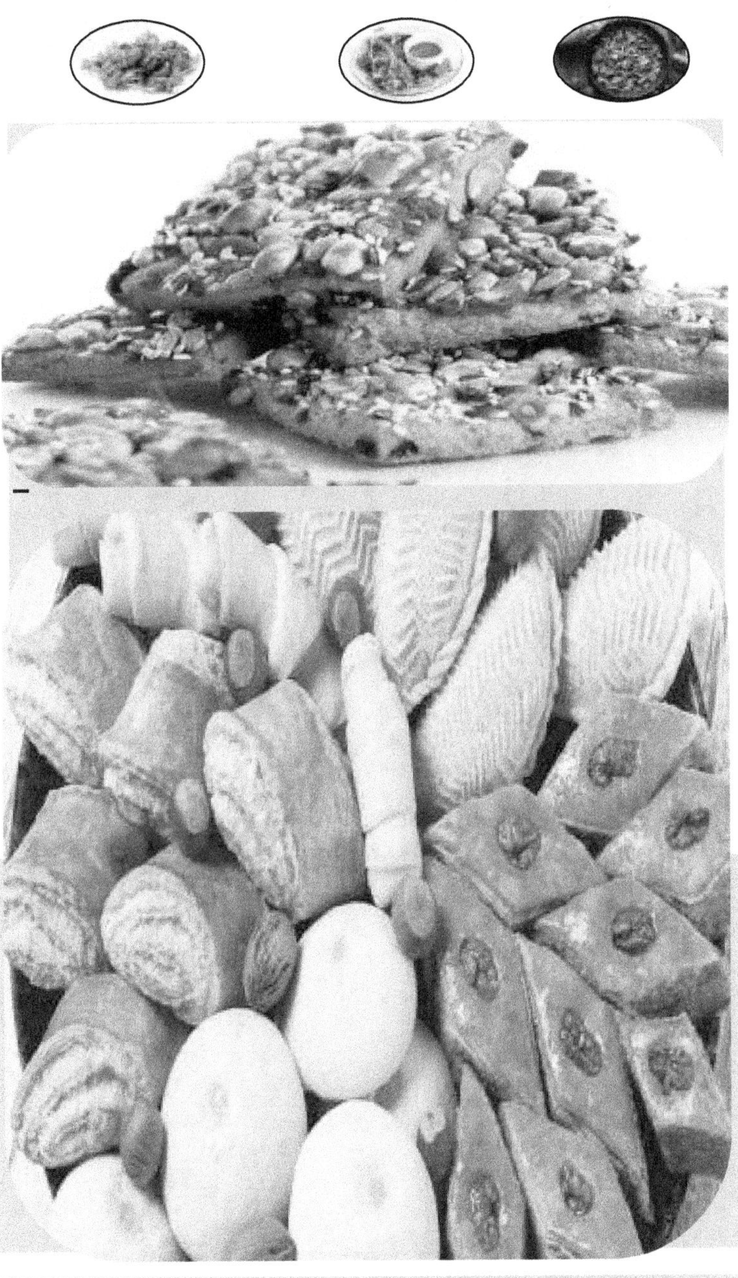

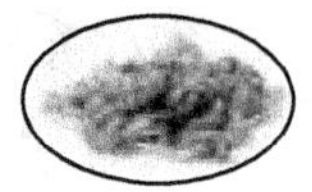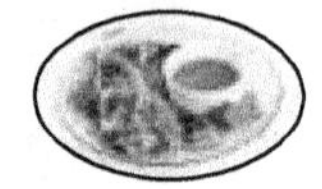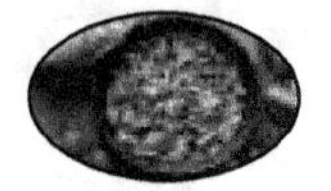

THAT'S WHY WE ARE SAYING THANK YOU...

"We know time is the unit of destiny, that's why we are saying thank you."

Dear Valued Customer,

we understand that time is a precious commodity, and we sincerely appreciate you choosing to spend a portion of it with us. Your decision to trust us with your purchase means the world to us, and we want to express our deepest gratitude.

Your support not only fuels our passion for delivering quality products but also contributes to the destiny of our business. Each customer is a vital part of our journey, and we are honored to have you

We strive to provide an exceptional shopping experience, and your satisfaction is our top priority. If you have any feedback or suggestions, we would love to hear from you. Your insights help us improve.

As a small token of our appreciation, we kindly invite you to share your experience by leaving a 5-star review. Your feedback not only boosts our morale but also assists fellow shoppers in making informed decisions.

Once again, thank you for choosing to buy this book. We look forward to serving you again and being a part of your destiny in the world of quality and excellence.

Warm regards,

Dr. Grace Hester–

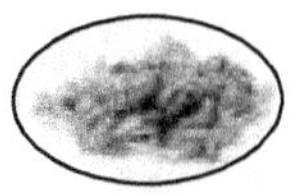
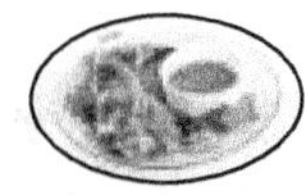
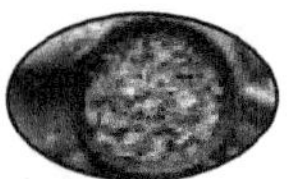

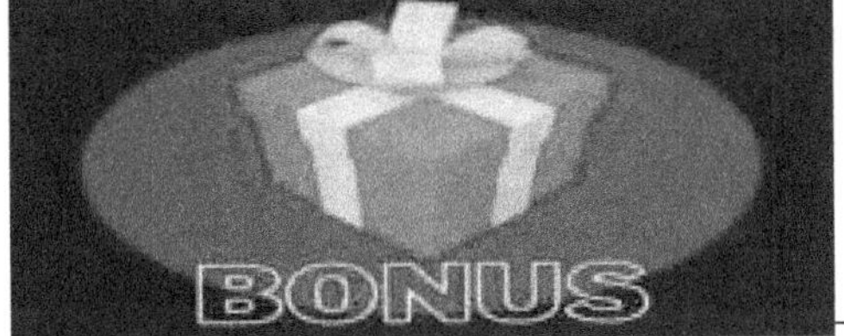

Gracehester.recipes@gmail.com–

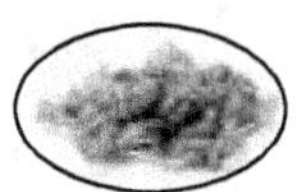 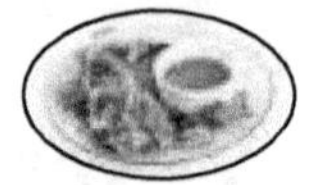 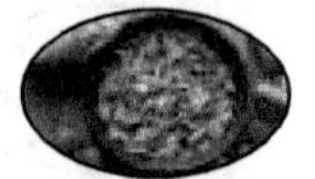

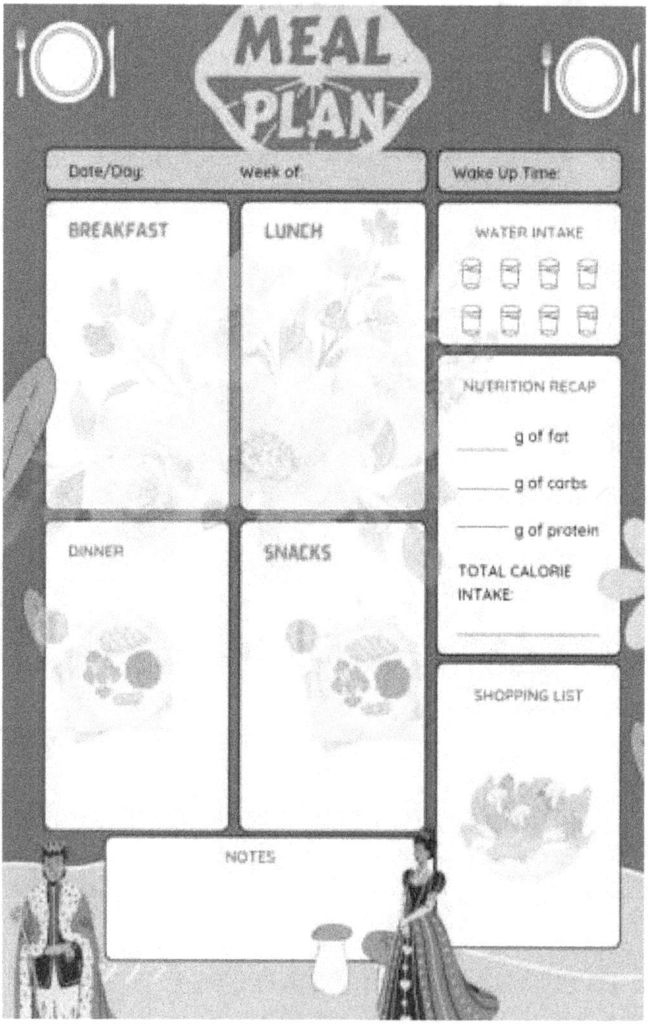

MEAL PLAN

| Date/Day: | Week of: | Wake Up Time: |

BREAKFAST

LUNCH

WATER INTAKE

NUTRITION RECAP

_______ g of fat

_______ g of carbs

_______ g of protein

TOTAL CALORIE INTAKE:

DINNER

SNACKS

SHOPPING LIST

NOTES

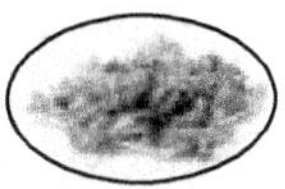 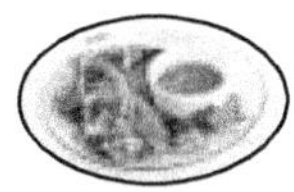 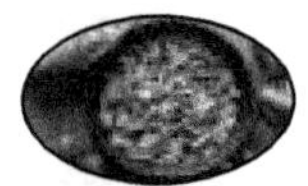

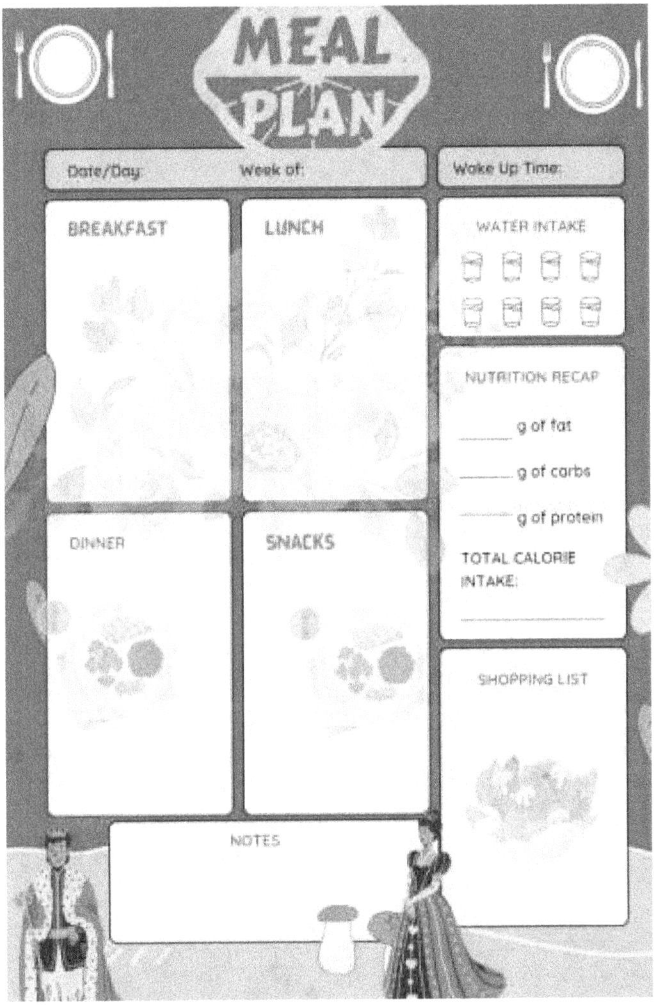

MEAL PLAN

| Date/Day: | Week of: | Wake Up Time: |

BREAKFAST

LUNCH

WATER INTAKE

NUTRITION RECAP

__________ g of fat

__________ g of carbs

__________ g of protein

TOTAL CALORIE INTAKE:

DINNER

SNACKS

SHOPPING LIST

NOTES

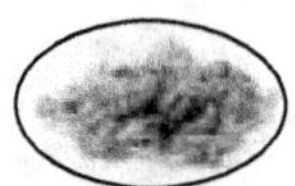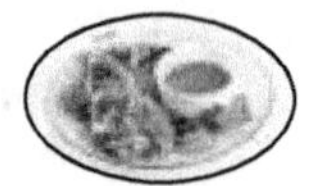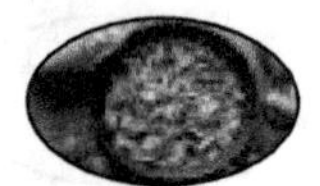

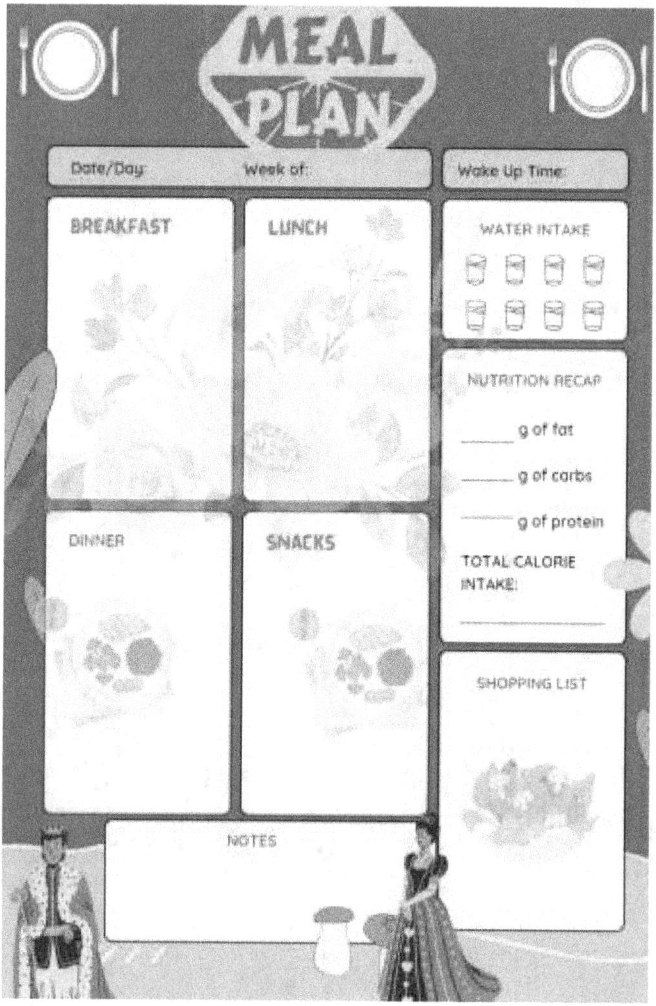

MEAL PLAN

Date/Day	Week of:	Wake Up Time:

BREAKFAST

LUNCH

WATER INTAKE

NUTRITION RECAP

__________ g of fat

__________ g of carbs

__________ g of protein

TOTAL CALORIE INTAKE:

____

DINNER

SNACKS

SHOPPING LIST

NOTES

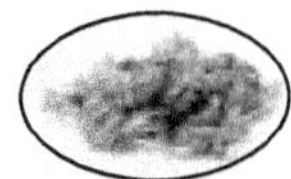 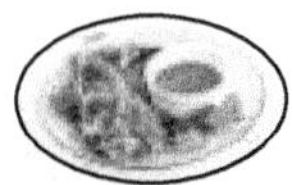 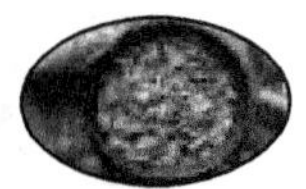

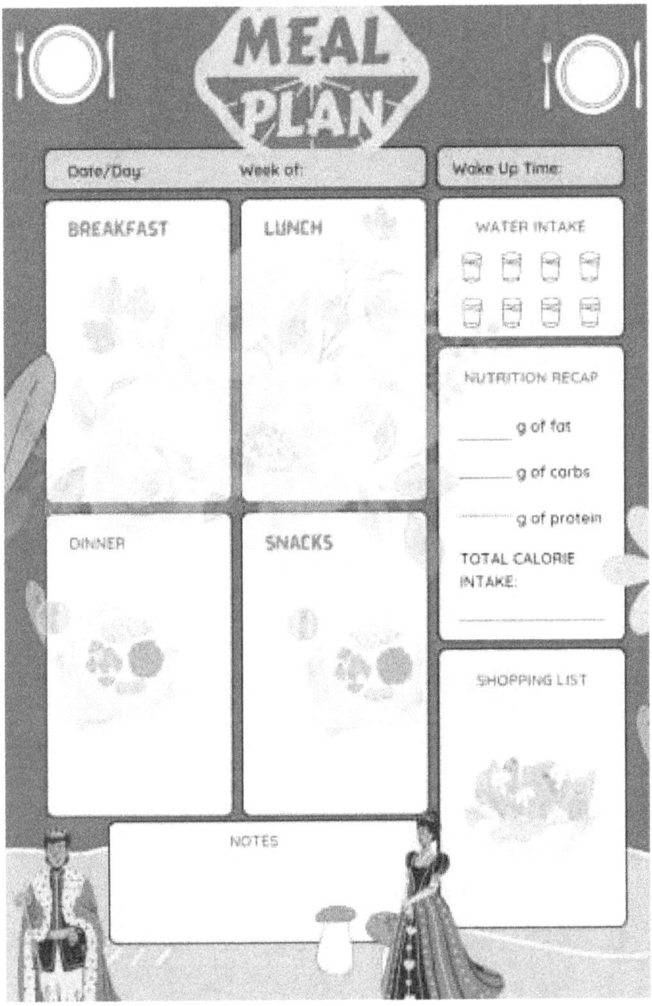

MEAL PLAN

| Date/Day | Week of: | Wake Up Time: |

BREAKFAST

LUNCH

WATER INTAKE

NUTRITION RECAP

__________ g of fat

__________ g of carbs

__________ g of protein

TOTAL CALORIE INTAKE:

DINNER

SNACKS

SHOPPING LIST

NOTES

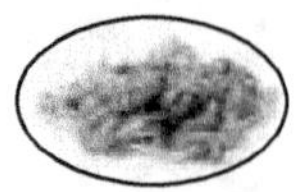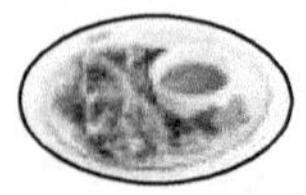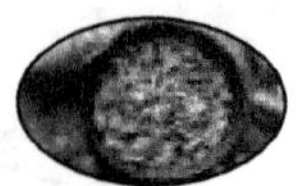

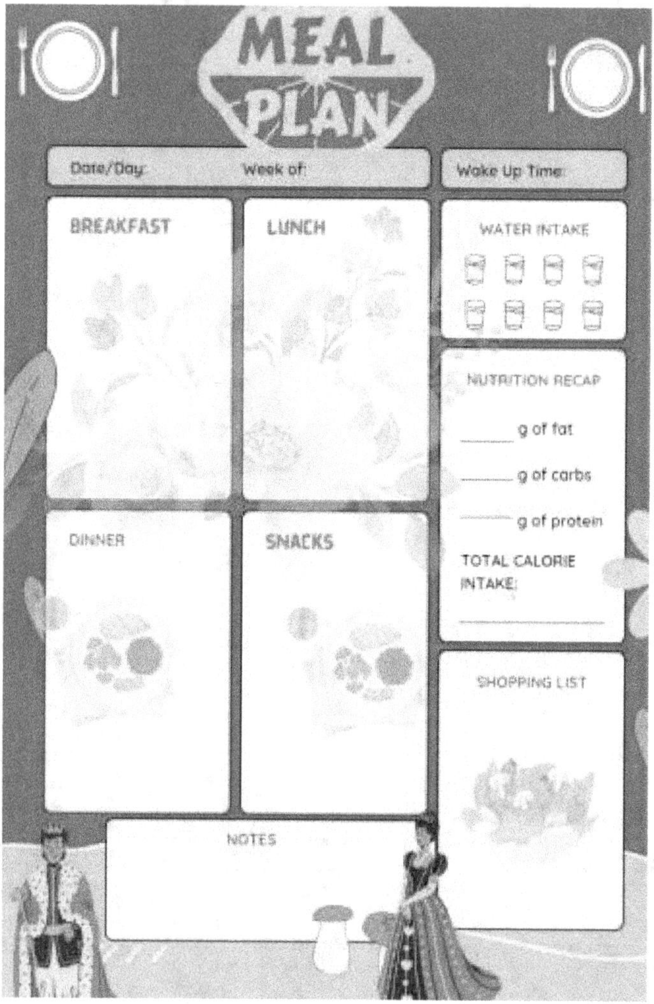

MEAL PLAN

| Date/Day: | Week of: | Wake Up Time: |

BREAKFAST

LUNCH

WATER INTAKE

NUTRITION RECAP

_____ g of fat

_____ g of carbs

_____ g of protein

TOTAL CALORIE INTAKE:

____

DINNER

SNACKS

SHOPPING LIST

NOTES

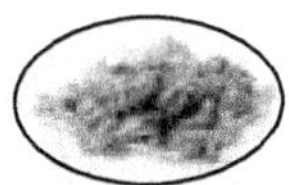
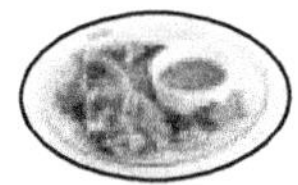
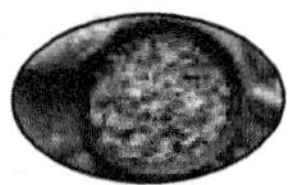

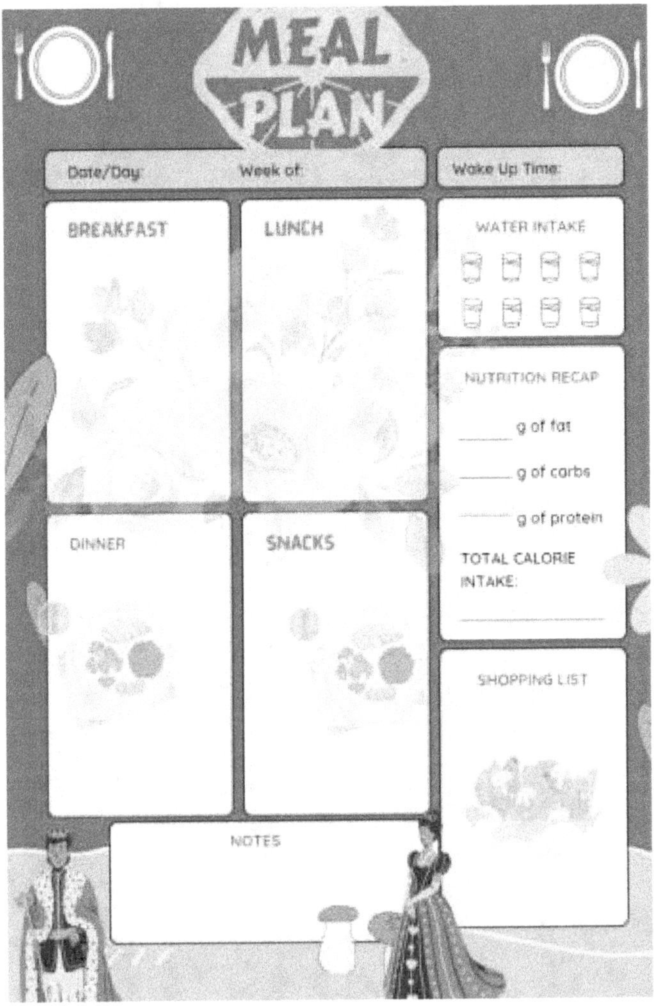

MEAL PLAN

| Date/Day: | Week of: | Wake Up Time: |

BREAKFAST

LUNCH

WATER INTAKE

DINNER

SNACKS

NUTRITION RECAP

__________ g of fat

__________ g of carbs

__________ g of protein

TOTAL CALORIE
INTAKE:

____

SHOPPING LIST

NOTES

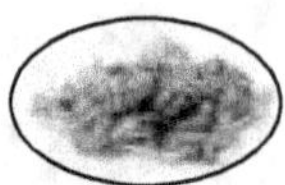
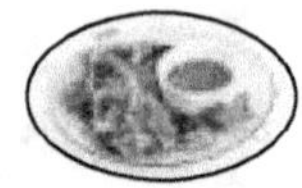
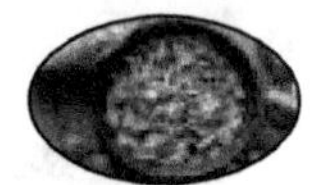

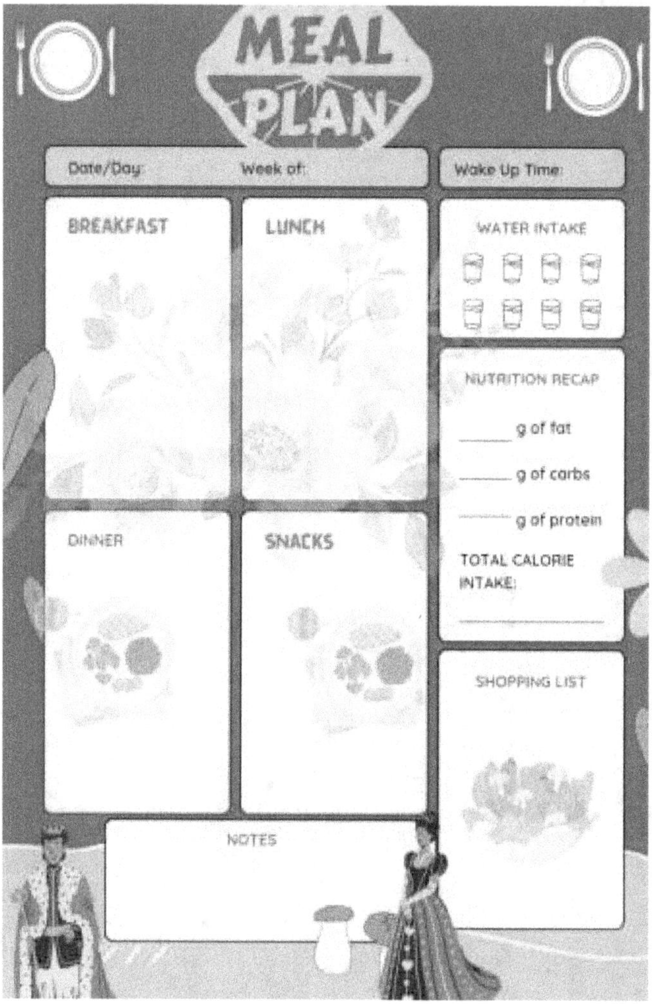

MEAL PLAN

Date/Day: Week of: Wake Up Time:

BREAKFAST

LUNCH

WATER INTAKE

NUTRITION RECAP

__________ g of fat

__________ g of carbs

__________ g of protein

TOTAL CALORIE INTAKE:

____

DINNER

SNACKS

SHOPPING LIST

NOTES

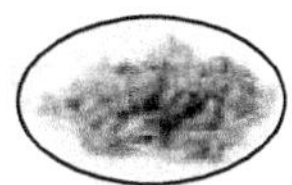 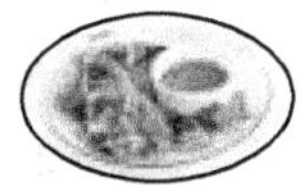 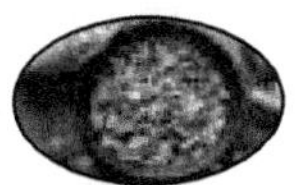

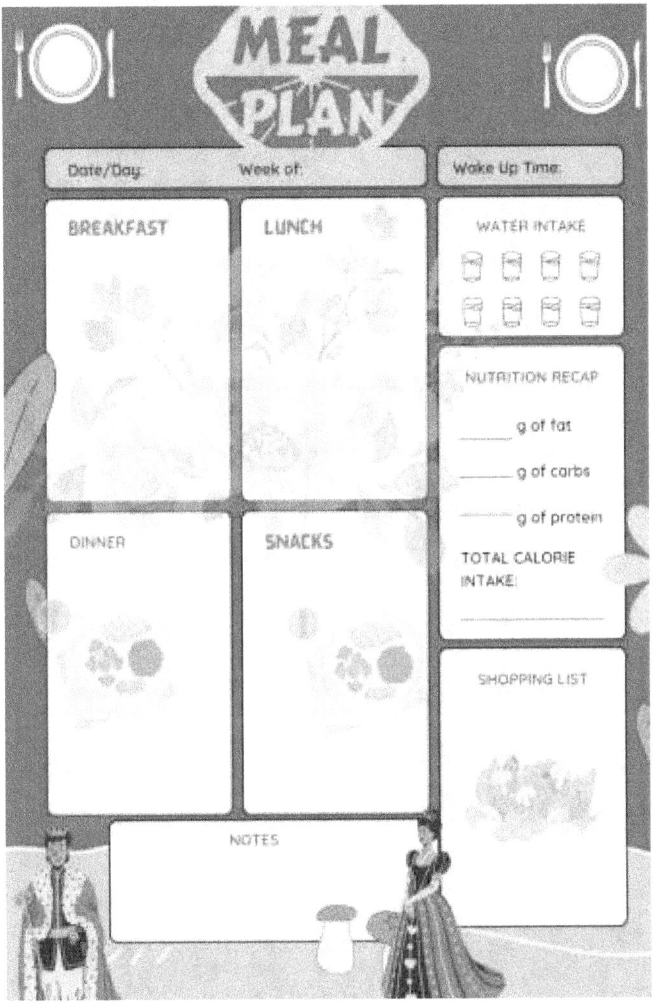

MEAL PLAN

| Date/Day: | Week of: | Woke Up Time: |

BREAKFAST

LUNCH

WATER INTAKE

NUTRITION RECAP

_________ g of fat

_________ g of carbs

_________ g of protein

TOTAL CALORIE INTAKE:

____

DINNER

SNACKS

SHOPPING LIST

NOTES

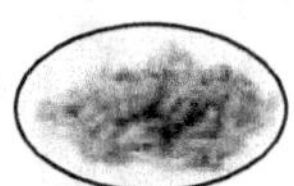 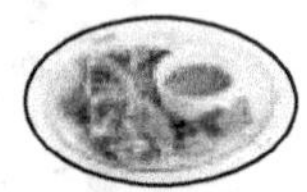 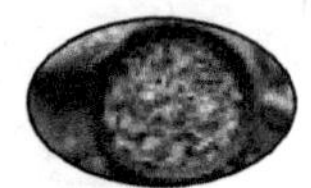

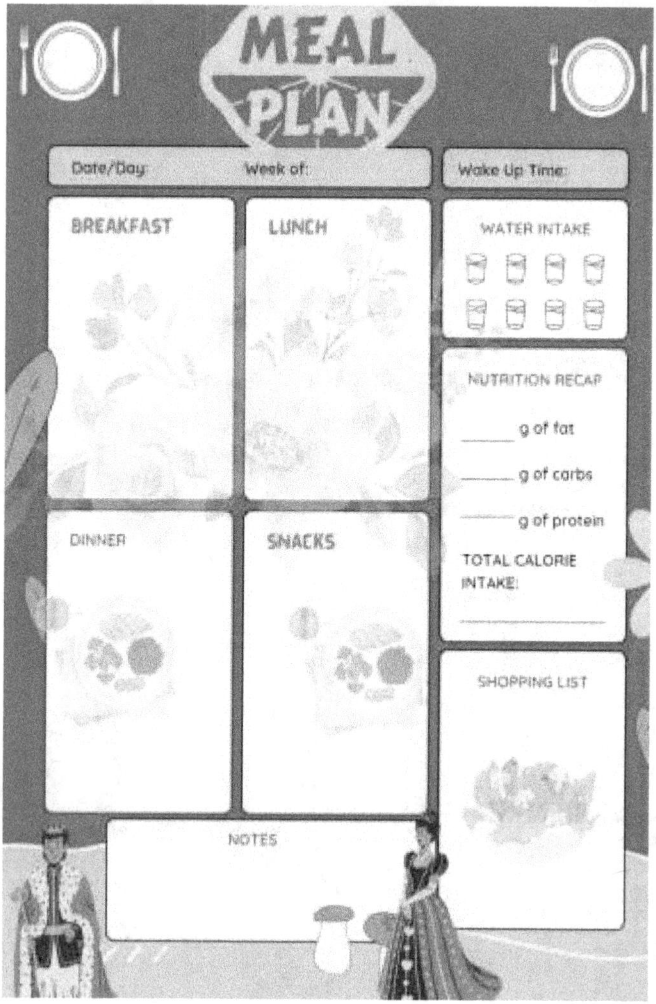

MEAL PLAN

| Date/Day: | Week of: | Wake Up Time: |

BREAKFAST

LUNCH

WATER INTAKE

NUTRITION RECAP

__________ g of fat

__________ g of carbs

__________ g of protein

TOTAL CALORIE INTAKE:

____

DINNER

SNACKS

SHOPPING LIST

NOTES

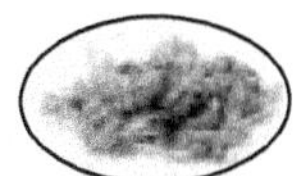 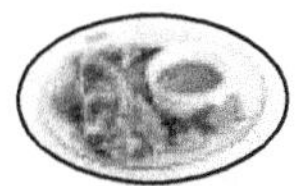 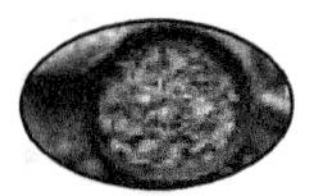

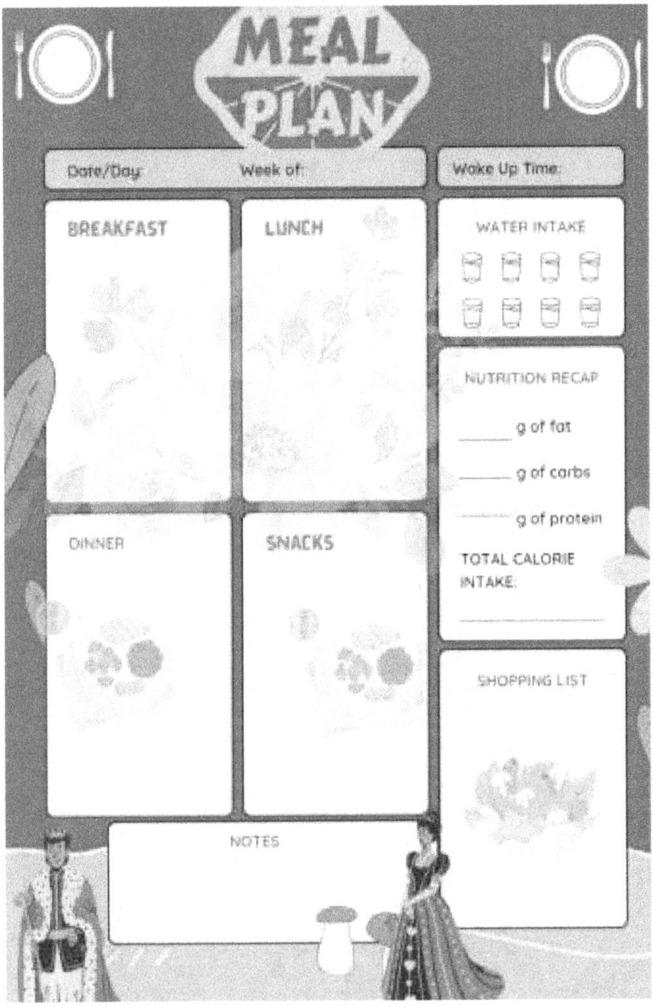

MEAL PLAN

| Date/Day: | Week of: | Wake Up Time: |

BREAKFAST

LUNCH

WATER INTAKE

NUTRITION RECAP

__________ g of fat

__________ g of carbs

__________ g of protein

TOTAL CALORIE INTAKE:

____

DINNER

SNACKS

SHOPPING LIST

NOTES

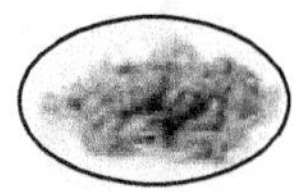 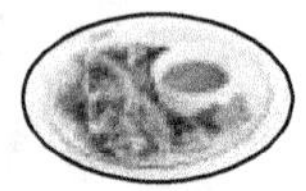 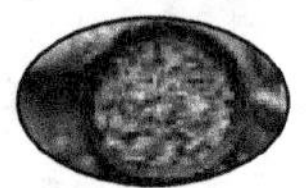

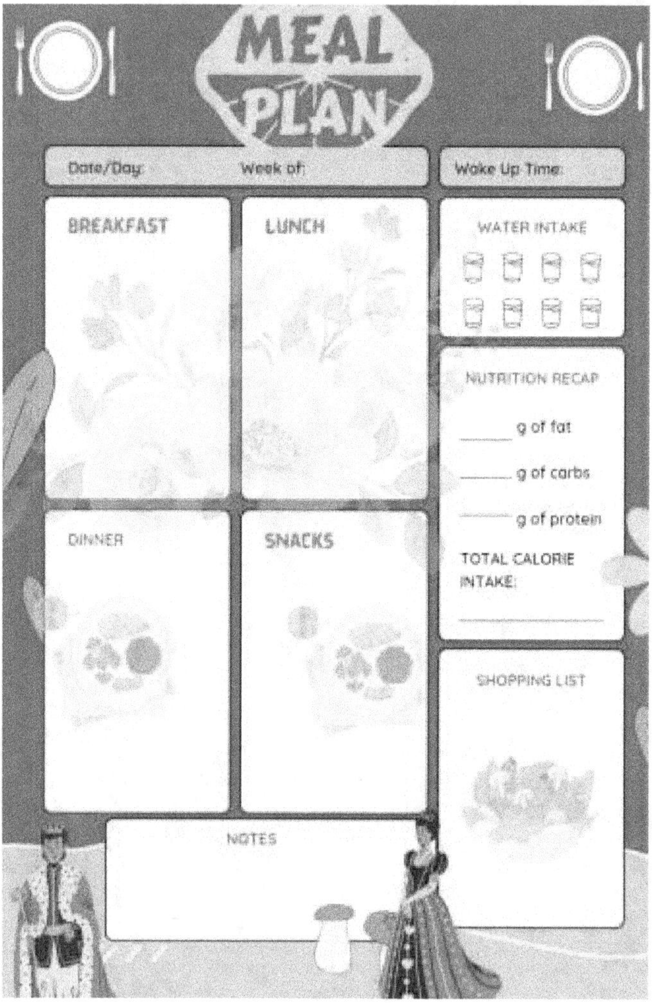

MEAL PLAN

| Date/Day: | Week of: | Wake Up Time: |

BREAKFAST

LUNCH

WATER INTAKE

NUTRITION RECAP

_______ g of fat

_______ g of carbs

_______ g of protein

TOTAL CALORIE INTAKE:

____

DINNER

SNACKS

SHOPPING LIST

NOTES

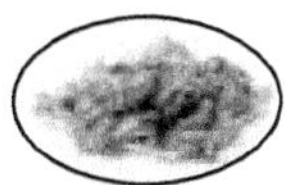 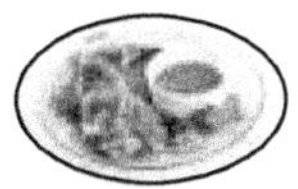 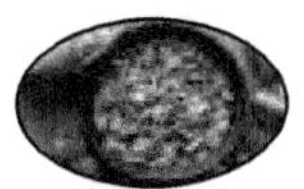

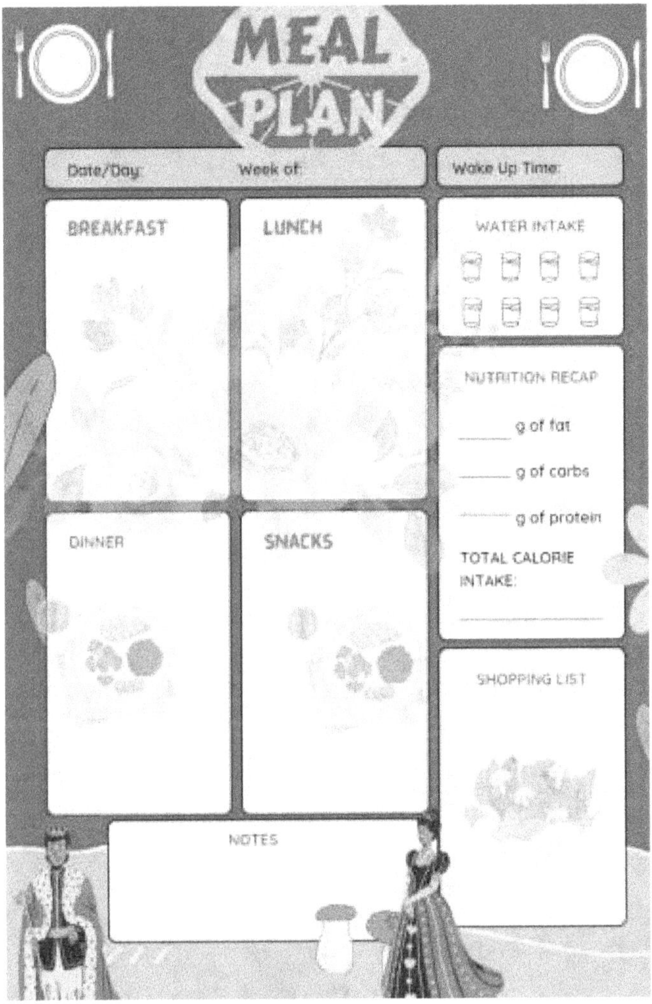

MEAL PLAN

| Date/Day: | Week of: | Wake Up Time: |

BREAKFAST

LUNCH

WATER INTAKE

NUTRITION RECAP

__________ g of fat

__________ g of carbs

__________ g of protein

TOTAL CALORIE INTAKE:

____

DINNER

SNACKS

SHOPPING LIST

NOTES

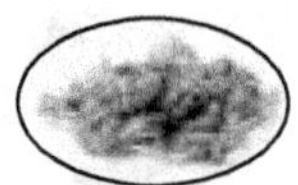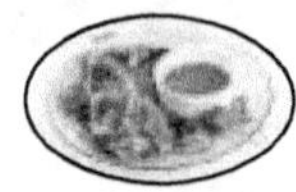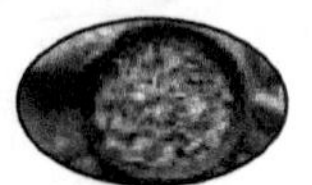

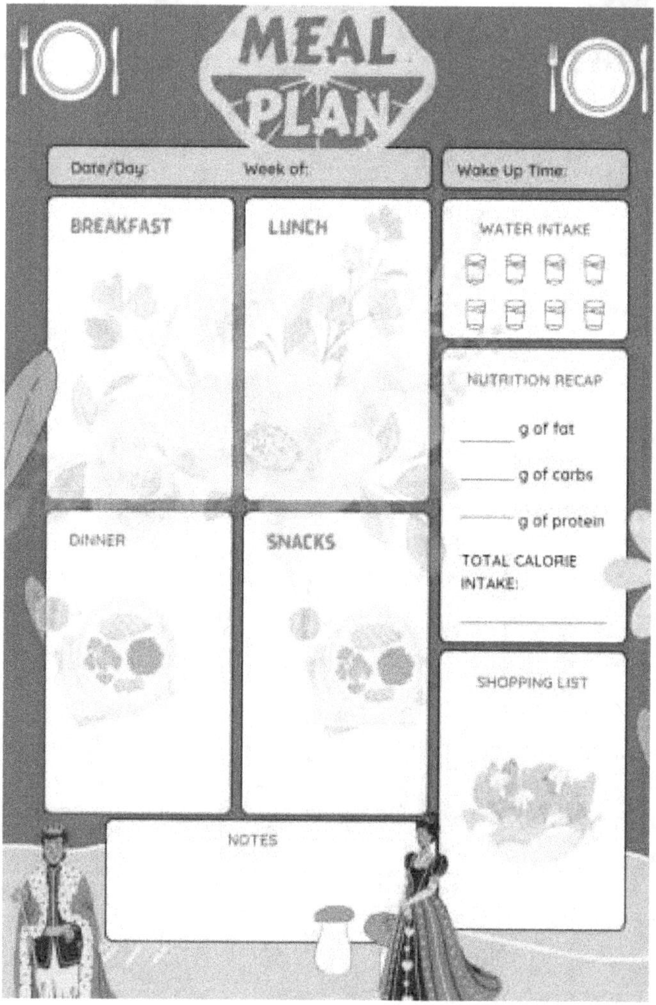

MEAL PLAN

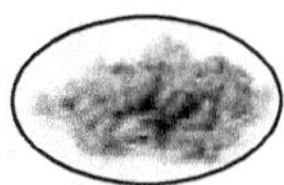 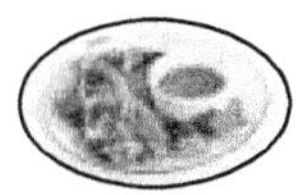 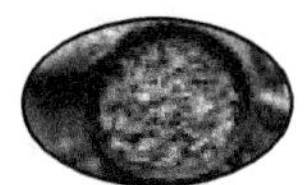

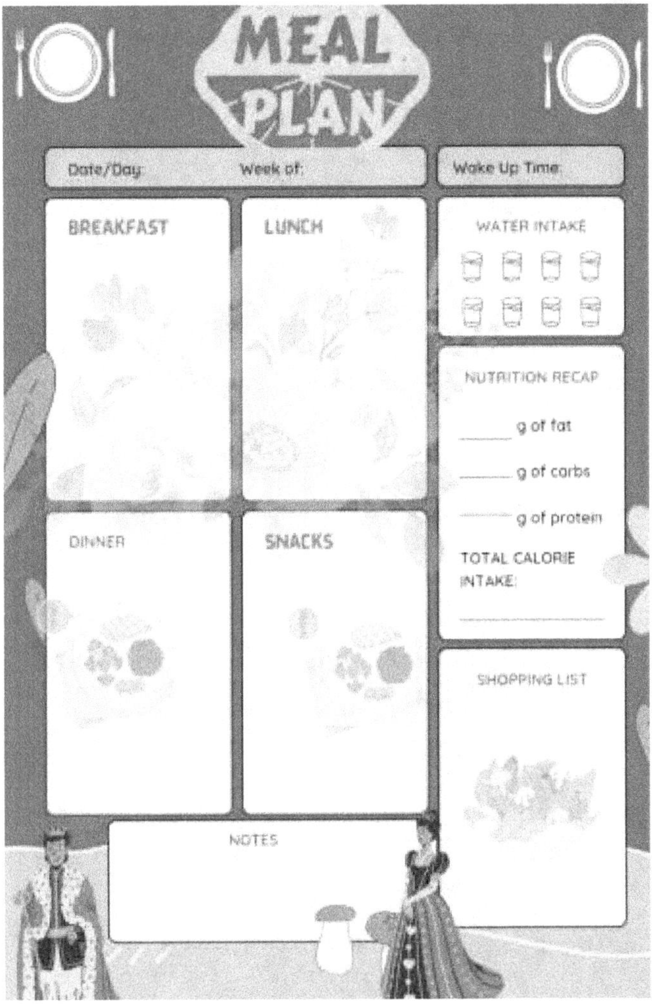

MEAL PLAN

| Date/Day: | Week of: | Wake Up Time: |

BREAKFAST

LUNCH

WATER INTAKE

NUTRITION RECAP

___________ g of fat

___________ g of carbs

___________ g of protein

TOTAL CALORIE INTAKE:

DINNER

SNACKS

SHOPPING LIST

NOTES

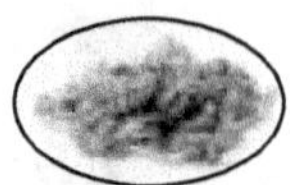 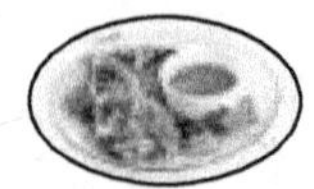 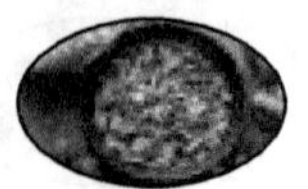

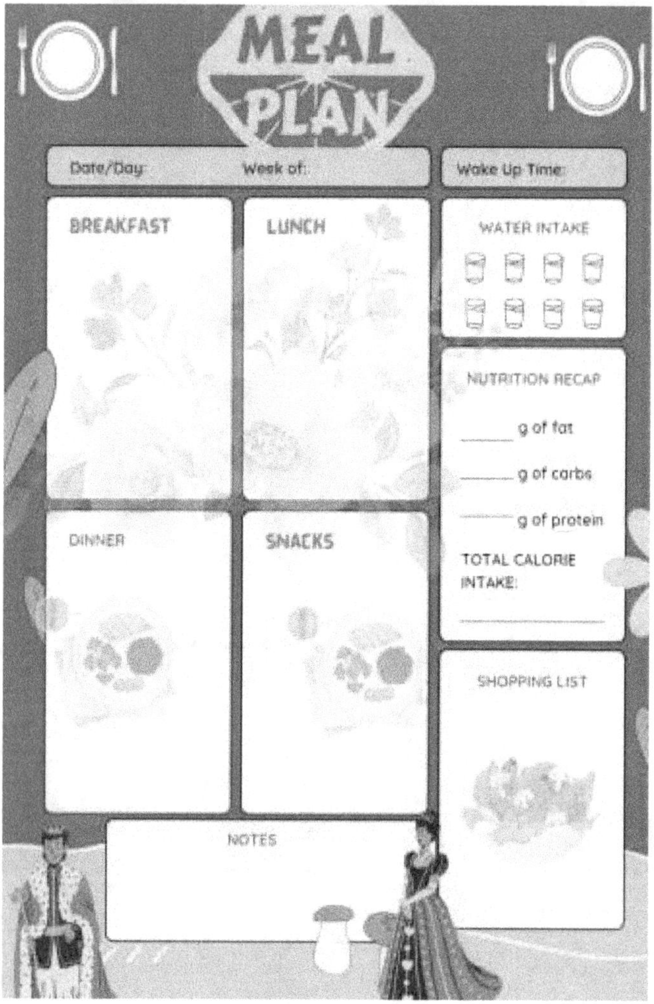

MEAL PLAN

Date/Day:	Week of:	Wake Up Time:

BREAKFAST

LUNCH

WATER INTAKE

NUTRITION RECAP

__________ g of fat

__________ g of carbs

__________ g of protein

TOTAL CALORIE INTAKE:

DINNER

SNACKS

SHOPPING LIST

NOTES

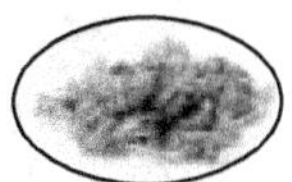 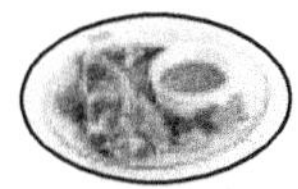 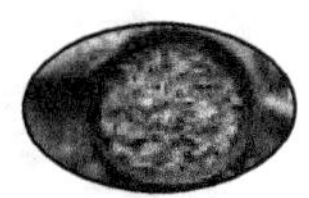

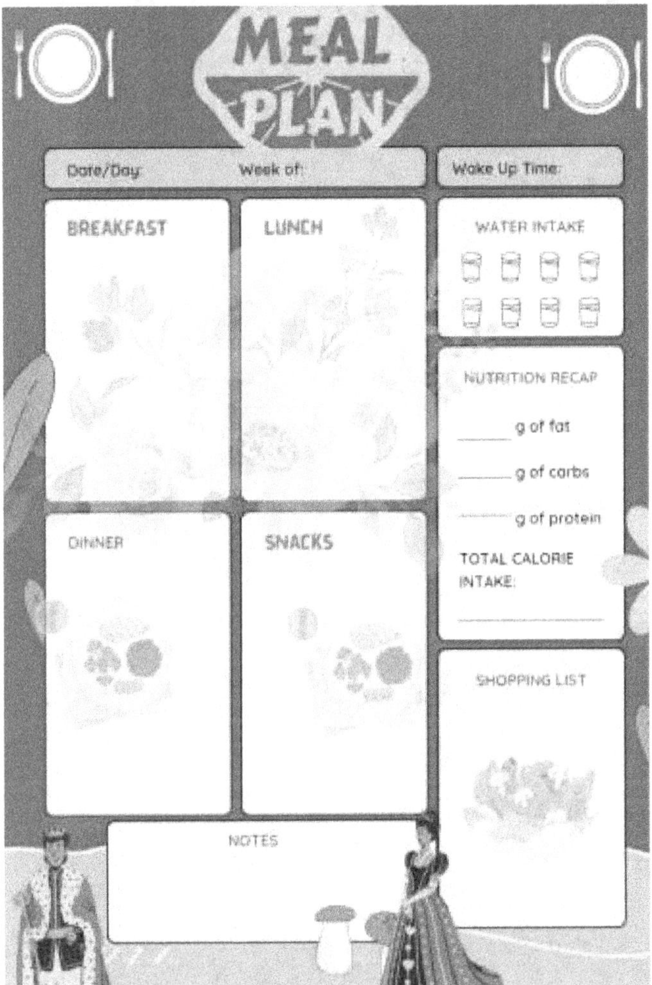

MEAL PLAN

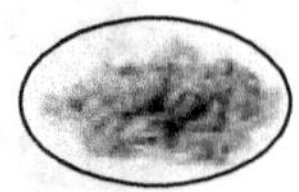 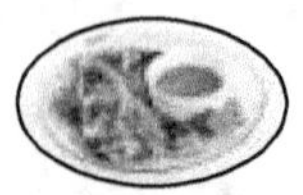 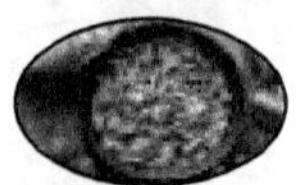

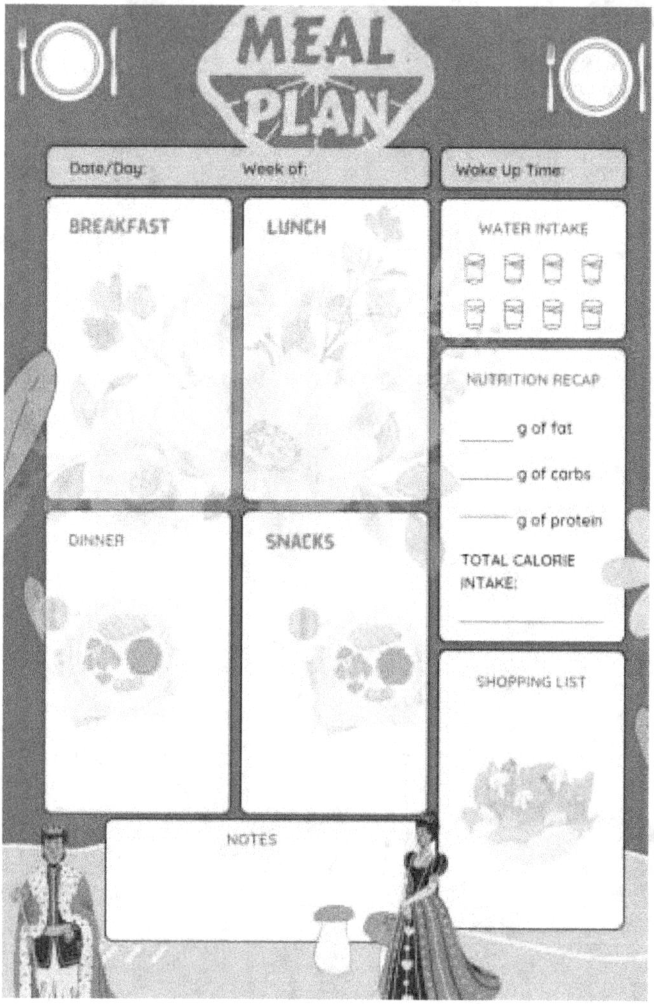

MEAL PLAN

| Date/Day: | Week of: | Woke Up Time: |

BREAKFAST

LUNCH

WATER INTAKE

NUTRITION RECAP

__________ g of fat

__________ g of carbs

__________ g of protein

TOTAL CALORIE INTAKE:

____

DINNER

SNACKS

SHOPPING LIST

NOTES

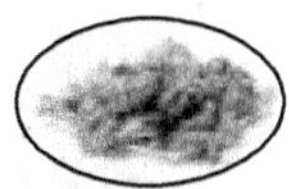
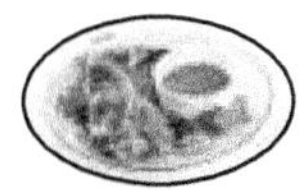
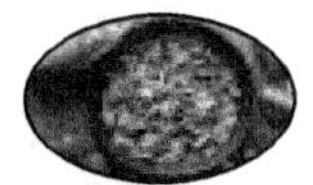

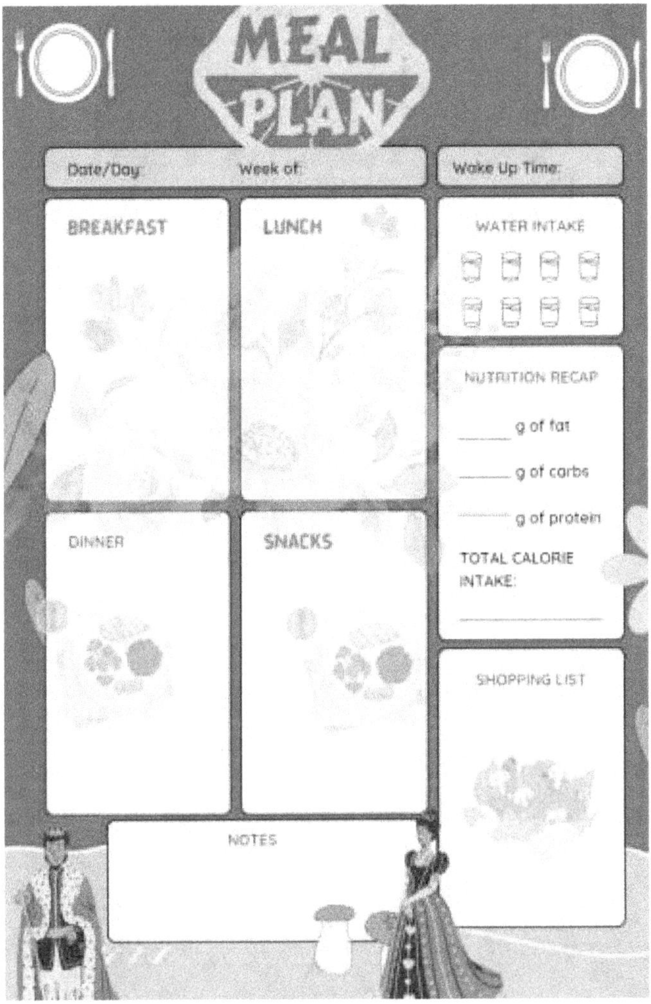

MEAL PLAN

Date/Day:	Week of:	Wake Up Time:

BREAKFAST

LUNCH

WATER INTAKE

NUTRITION RECAP

__________ g of fat

__________ g of carbs

__________ g of protein

TOTAL CALORIE INTAKE:

____

DINNER

SNACKS

SHOPPING LIST

NOTES

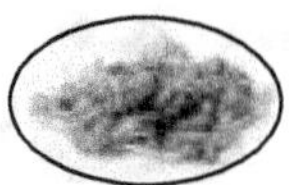 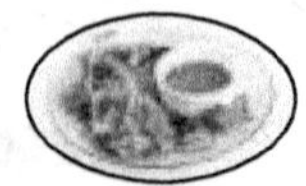 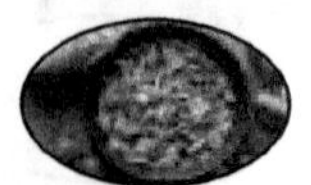

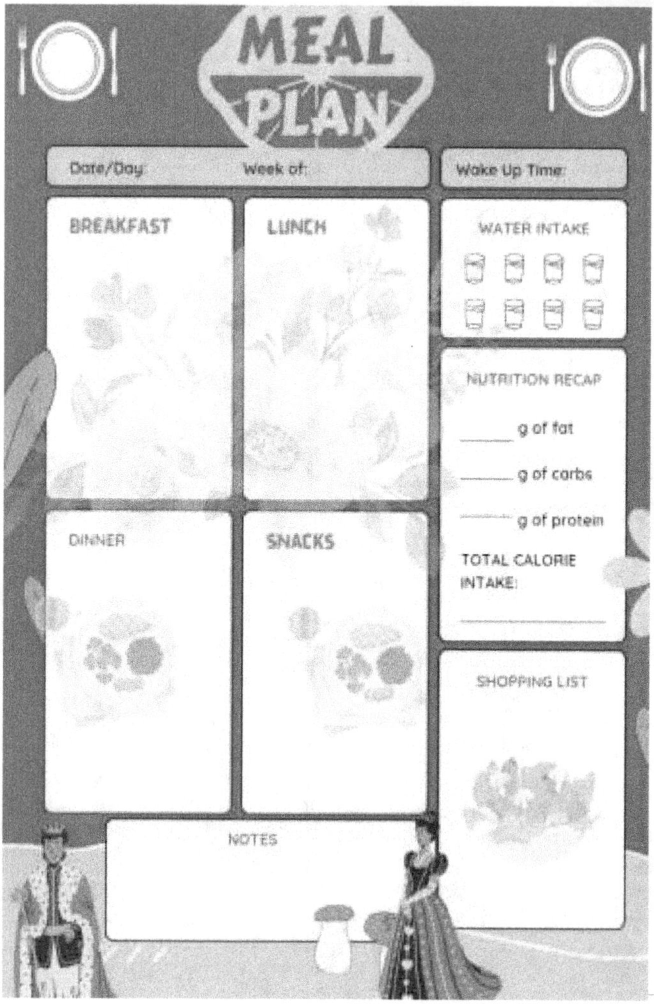

MEAL PLAN

Date/Day:	Week of:	Wake Up Time:

BREAKFAST

LUNCH

WATER INTAKE

NUTRITION RECAP

__________ g of fat

__________ g of carbs

__________ g of protein

TOTAL CALORIE INTAKE:

____

DINNER

SNACKS

SHOPPING LIST

NOTES

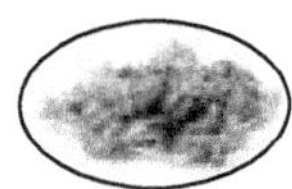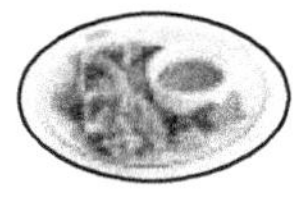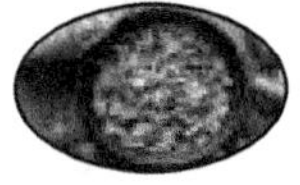

We are sure you enjoyed reading this straight to the point book, to get more on Dr. Grace Hester, scan the QR code below;

www.ingramcontent.com/pod-product-compliance
Lightning Source LLC
Chambersburg PA
CBHW061010260726
48661CB00005B/2150